P9-DME-456

STRENGTH TRAINING
ANATOMY

FRÉDÉRIC DELAVIER

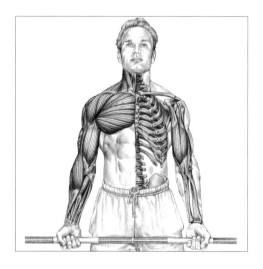

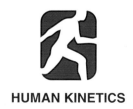

HUMAN KINETICS

Library of Congress Cataloging-in-Publication Data

Delavier, Frédéric.
    Strength training anatomy / Frédéric Delavier.
        p. cm.
    Rev. ed. of: Guide des mouvements de musculation. Paris: Éditions Vigot, 1998.
    ISBN 0-7360-4185-0
    1. Muscles--Anatomy. 2. Weight training. 3. Muscle strength. I. Delavier, Frédéric.
Guide des mouvements de musculation. II. Title.

    QM151 .D454 2001
    611'.73--dc21   2001024513

ISBN: 0-7360-4185-0

Copyright © 2001 by Éditions Vigot – 23, rue de l'École-de-Médecine, 75006 Paris, France.

All rights reserved. Except for use in a review, the reproduction or utilization of this work in any form or by any electronic, mechanical, or other means, now known or hereafter invented, including xerography, photocopying, and recording, and in any information storage and retrieval system, is forbidden without the written permission of the publisher.

This book is a revised edition of Guide des Mouvements de Musculation, published in 1998 by Éditions Vigot.

Acquisitions Editor: Martin Barnard
Managing Editor: Stephan Seyfert
Translators: G. Hubert, P. Gross, and Robert H. Black R.M.T.
Copyeditor: Karen L. Marker
Cover Designer: Keith Blomberg
Illustrator: Frédéric Delavier

Human Kinetics books are available at special discounts for bulk purchase. Special editions or book excerpts can also be created to specification. For details, contact the Special Sales Manager at Human Kinetics.

Printed in France by Pollina, n° L89549   10 9

Human Kinetics
Web site: www.humankinetics.com

United States: Human Kinetics
P.O. Box 5076
Champaign, IL 61825-5076
800-747-4457
e-mail: humank@hkusa.com

Canada: Human Kinetics
475 Devonshire Road Unit 100
Windsor, ON N8Y 2L5
800-465-7301 (in Canada only)
e-mail: orders@hkcanada.com

Europe: Human Kinetics
107 Bradford Road
Stanningley
Leeds LS28 6AT, United Kingdom
+44 (0)113 255 5665
e-mail: hk@hkeurope.com

Australia: Human Kinetics
57A Price Avenue
Lower Mitcham, South Australia 5062
08 8277 1555
e-mail: liahka@senet.com.au

New Zealand: Human Kinetics
P.O. Box 105-231, Auckland Central
09-523-3462
e-mail: hkp@ihug.co.nz

for my father

CONTENTS

1 ARMS

1. Curls
2. Concentration Curls
3. Hammer Curls
4. Low Pulley Curls
5. High Pulley Curls
6. Barbell Curls
7. Machine Curls
8. Preacher Curls
9. Reverse Curls
10. Reverse Wrist Curls
11. Wrist Curls
12. Pushdowns
13. Reverse Pushdowns
14. One-Arm Reverse Pushdowns
15. Triceps Extensions
16. Dumbbell Triceps Extensions
17. One-Arm Dumbbell Triceps Extensions
18. Seated Dumbbell Triceps Extensions
19. Seated EZ-Bar Triceps Extensions
20. Triceps Kickbacks
21. Triceps Dips

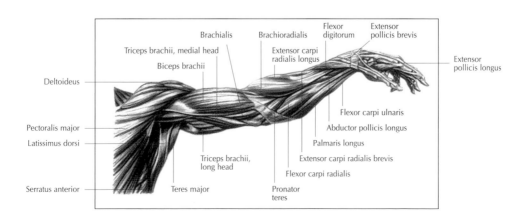

1 CURLS

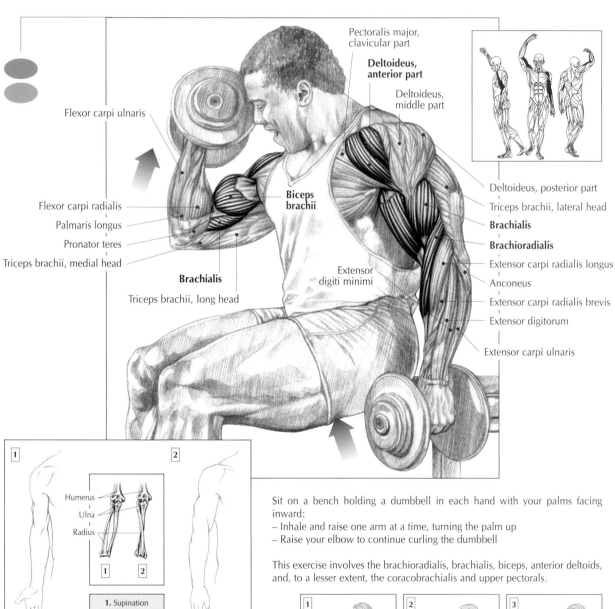

Flexor carpi ulnaris

Flexor carpi radialis
Palmaris longus
Pronator teres
Triceps brachii, medial head

Biceps brachii

Brachialis
Triceps brachii, long head

Pectoralis major, clavicular part
Deltoideus, anterior part
Deltoideus, middle part

Extensor digiti minimi

Deltoideus, posterior part
Triceps brachii, lateral head
Brachialis
Brachioradialis
Extensor carpi radialis longus
Anconeus
Extensor carpi radialis brevis
Extensor digitorum
Extensor carpi ulnaris

Humerus
Ulna
Radius

1. Supination
2. Pronation

Sit on a bench holding a dumbbell in each hand with your palms facing inward:
– Inhale and raise one arm at a time, turning the palm up
– Raise your elbow to continue curling the dumbbell

This exercise involves the brachioradialis, brachialis, biceps, anterior deltoids, and, to a lesser extent, the coracobrachialis and upper pectorals.

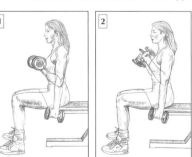
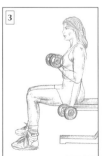

Note: biomechanically, this exercise is excellent for emphasizing the biceps in all its actions (flexion and protraction of the arm and supination).

THREE WAYS TO CURL DUMBBELLS:
1. work both the biceps and brachialis
2. mainly work the brachioradialis
3. mainly work the biceps

CONCENTRATION CURLS 2

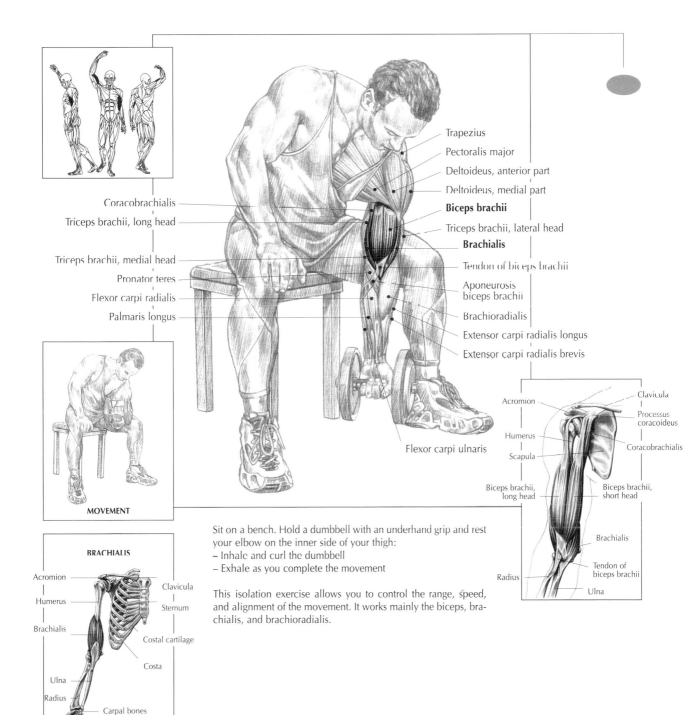

Coracobrachialis
Triceps brachii, long head

Triceps brachii, medial head
Pronator teres
Flexor carpi radialis
Palmaris longus

Trapezius
Pectoralis major
Deltoideus, anterior part
Deltoideus, medial part
Biceps brachii
Triceps brachii, lateral head
Brachialis
Tendon of biceps brachii
Aponeurosis biceps brachii
Brachioradialis
Extensor carpi radialis longus
Extensor carpi radialis brevis

Flexor carpi ulnaris

MOVEMENT

BRACHIALIS

Acromion
Humerus
Brachialis
Ulna
Radius
acarpal bones
iddle phalanx

Clavicula
Sternum
Costal cartilage
Costa
Carpal bones
Proximal phalanx
Distal phalanx

Acromion
Humerus
Scapula
Biceps brachii, long head
Radius

Clavicula
Processus coracoideus
Coracobrachialis
Biceps brachii, short head
Brachialis
Tendon of biceps brachii
Ulna

Sit on a bench. Hold a dumbbell with an underhand grip and rest your elbow on the inner side of your thigh:
– Inhale and curl the dumbbell
– Exhale as you complete the movement

This isolation exercise allows you to control the range, speed, and alignment of the movement. It works mainly the biceps, brachialis, and brachioradialis.

3 HAMMER CURLS

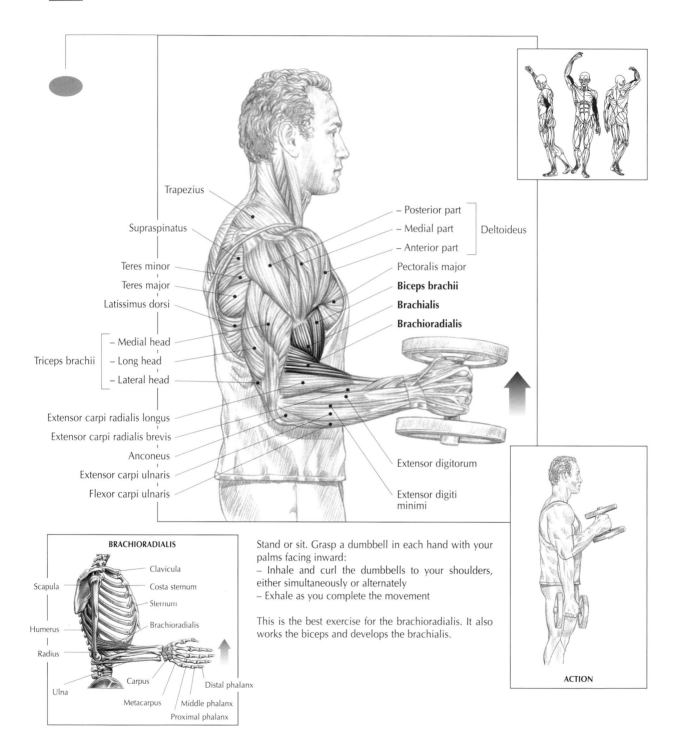

Trapezius

Supraspinatus

Teres minor

Teres major

Latissimus dorsi

Triceps brachii
– Medial head
– Long head
– Lateral head

Extensor carpi radialis longus

Extensor carpi radialis brevis

Anconeus

Extensor carpi ulnaris

Flexor carpi ulnaris

– Posterior part
– Medial part
– Anterior part
Deltoideus

Pectoralis major

Biceps brachii

Brachialis

Brachioradialis

Extensor digitorum

Extensor digiti minimi

BRACHIORADIALIS

Clavicula

Costa sternum

Sternum

Brachioradialis

Scapula

Humerus

Radius

Ulna

Carpus

Metacarpus

Proximal phalanx

Middle phalanx

Distal phalanx

Stand or sit. Grasp a dumbbell in each hand with your palms facing inward:
– Inhale and curl the dumbbells to your shoulders, either simultaneously or alternately
– Exhale as you complete the movement

This is the best exercise for the brachioradialis. It also works the biceps and develops the brachialis.

ACTION

LOW PULLEY CURLS 4

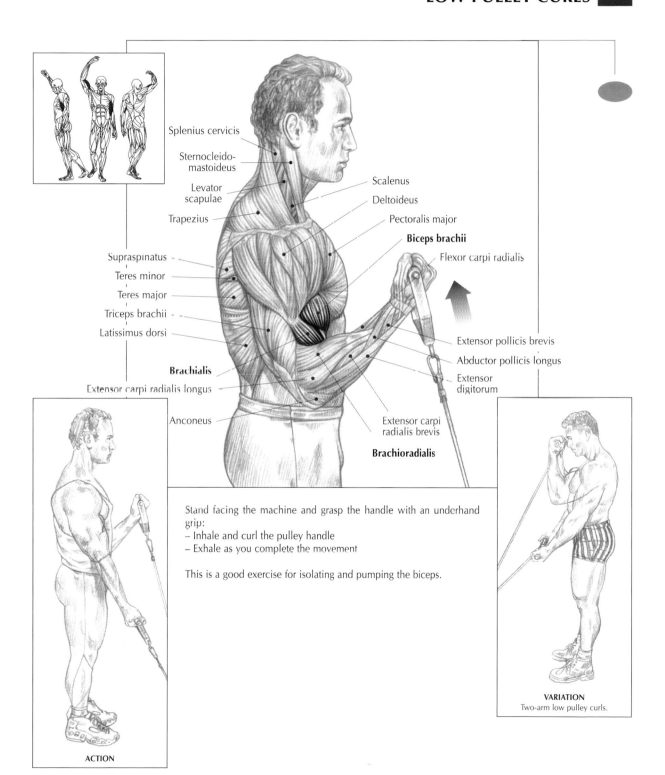

Splenius cervicis

Sternocleido-mastoideus

Levator scapulae

Trapezius

Scalenus

Deltoideus

Pectoralis major

Biceps brachii

Flexor carpi radialis

Supraspinatus

Teres minor

Teres major

Triceps brachii

Latissimus dorsi

Brachialis

Extensor carpi radialis longus

Anconeus

Extensor pollicis brevis

Abductor pollicis longus

Extensor digitorum

Extensor carpi radialis brevis

Brachioradialis

Stand facing the machine and grasp the handle with an underhand grip:
– Inhale and curl the pulley handle
– Exhale as you complete the movement

This is a good exercise for isolating and pumping the biceps.

VARIATION
Two-arm low pulley curls.

ACTION

5 HIGH PULLEY CURLS

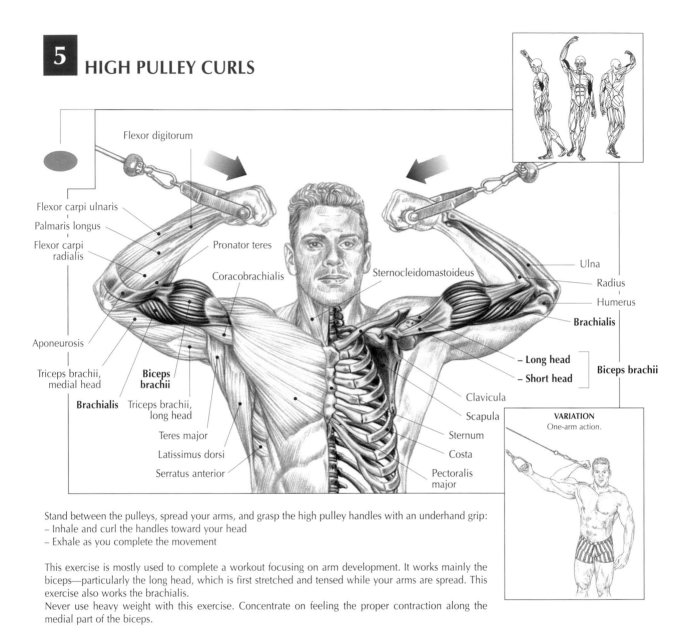

Flexor digitorum

Flexor carpi ulnaris

Palmaris longus

Flexor carpi radialis

Pronator teres

Coracobrachialis

Sternocleidomastoideus

Ulna

Radius

Humerus

Brachialis

Aponeurosis

Triceps brachii, medial head

Biceps brachii

Brachialis

Triceps brachii, long head

Teres major

Latissimus dorsi

Serratus anterior

– Long head

– Short head

Biceps brachii

Clavicula

Scapula

Sternum

Costa

Pectoralis major

VARIATION
One-arm action.

Stand between the pulleys, spread your arms, and grasp the high pulley handles with an underhand grip:
– Inhale and curl the handles toward your head
– Exhale as you complete the movement

This exercise is mostly used to complete a workout focusing on arm development. It works mainly the biceps—particularly the long head, which is first stretched and tensed while your arms are spread. This exercise also works the brachialis.
Never use heavy weight with this exercise. Concentrate on feeling the proper contraction along the medial part of the biceps.

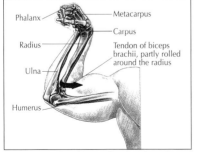

Phalanx

Metacarpus

Carpus

Radius

Tendon of biceps brachii, partly rolled around the radius

Ulna

Humerus

With an overhand grip, the distal tendon of the biceps is partly rolled around the radius.

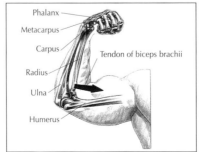

Phalanx

Metacarpus

Carpus

Radius

Tendon of biceps brachii

Ulna

Humerus

When you contract the biceps, the force exerted on its distal tendon rotates the radius around its axis, bringing the hand to a supinated position.

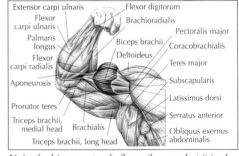

Extensor carpi ulnaris

Flexor carpi ulnaris

Palmaris longus

Flexor carpi radialis

Aponeurosis

Pronator teres

Triceps brachii, medial head

Triceps brachii, long head

Flexor digitorum

Brachioradialis

Pectoralis major

Biceps brachii

Coracobrachialis

Deltoideus

Teres major

Subscapularis

Latissimus dorsi

Serratus anterior

Obliquus exernus abdominalis

Brachialis

Note: the biceps not only flexes the arm, but it is also the most powerful supinator.

BARBELL CURLS 6

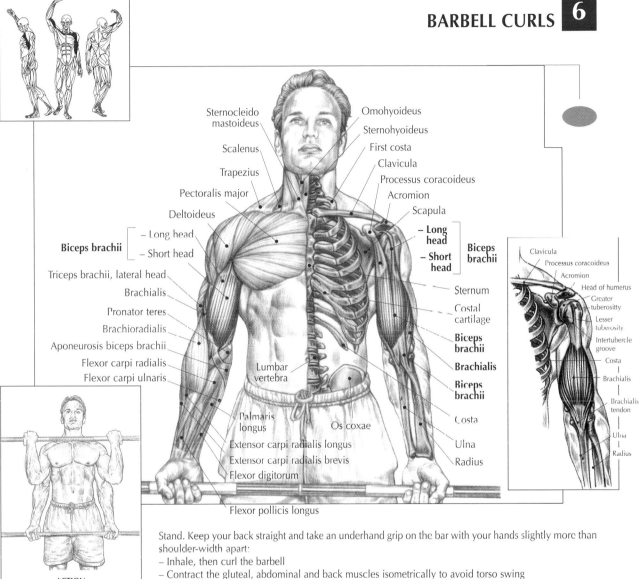

Sternocleido mastoideus
Scalenus
Trapezius
Pectoralis major
Deltoideus
Biceps brachii – Long head
– Short head
Triceps brachii, lateral head
Brachialis
Pronator teres
Brachioradialis
Aponeurosis biceps brachii
Flexor carpi radialis
Flexor carpi ulnaris
Palmaris longus
Extensor carpi radialis longus
Extensor carpi radialis brevis
Flexor digitorum
Flexor pollicis longus

Omohyoideus
Sternohyoideus
First costa
Clavicula
Processus coracoideus
Acromion
Scapula
Biceps brachii – **Long head**
– **Short head**
Sternum
Costal cartilage
Biceps brachii
Brachialis
Biceps brachii
Costa
Ulna
Radius
Lumbar vertebra
Os coxae

Clavicula
Processus coracoideus
Acromion
Head of humerus
Greater tuberositty
Lesser tuberosity
Intertubercle groove
Costa
Brachialis
Brachialis tendon
Ulna
Radius

ACTION

Stand. Keep your back straight and take an underhand grip on the bar with your hands slightly more than shoulder-width apart:
– Inhale, then curl the barbell
– Contract the gluteal, abdominal and back muscles isometrically to avoid torso swing
– Exhale as you complete the movement

This exercise mainly works the biceps, brachialis, and, to a lesser degree, the brachioradialis, pronator teres, and all the flexors of the wrist and fingers.

Variations:
1. Try using various grip widths to more intensely work
– the biceps short head (wide grip) or
– the biceps long head (narrow grip).
2. Lift your elbows at the end of the curl to get a better biceps contraction and to involve the anterior deltoids.
3. To make this movement more rigorous and controlled, place your back against a wall and keep your scapulae (shoulder blades) pressed against the wall.

VARIATIONS
Narrow grip: mainly works the biceps long head.
Wide grip: mainly works the biceps short head.

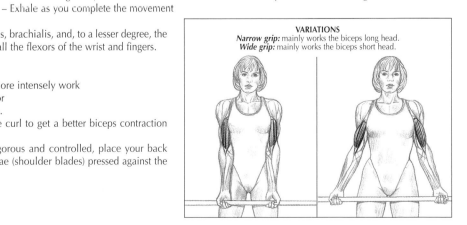

7 MACHINE CURLS

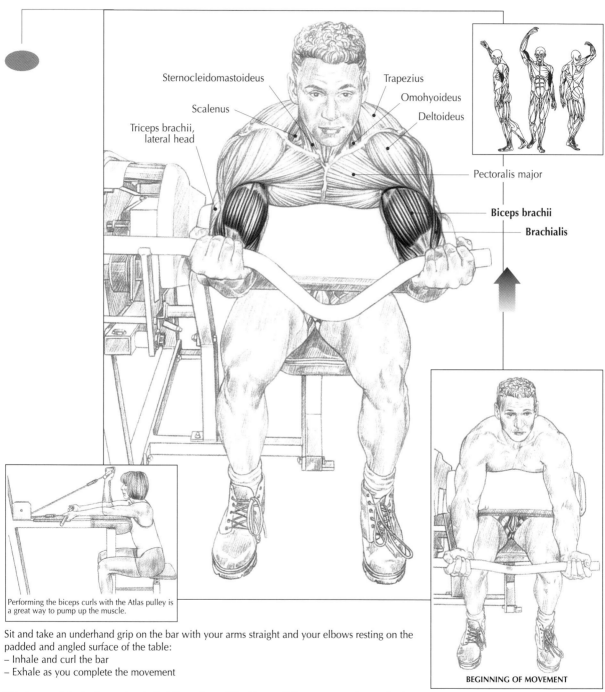

Sternocleidomastoideus

Scalenus

Triceps brachii,
lateral head

Trapezius

Omohyoideus

Deltoideus

Pectoralis major

Biceps brachii

Brachialis

Performing the biceps curls with the Atlas pulley is
a great way to pump up the muscle.

BEGINNING OF MOVEMENT

Sit and take an underhand grip on the bar with your arms straight and your elbows resting on the
padded and angled surface of the table:
– Inhale and curl the bar
– Exhale as you complete the movement

This is one of the best exercises to feel the action of the biceps. This movement also works the
brachialis and, to a lesser extent, the brachioradialis and pronator teres. It is impossible to cheat
because your arms are firmly held on the table. The muscular tension is intense at the beginning, so
warm up by using light loads. Avoid tendinitis by keeping your arms from extending completely.

PREACHER CURLS 8

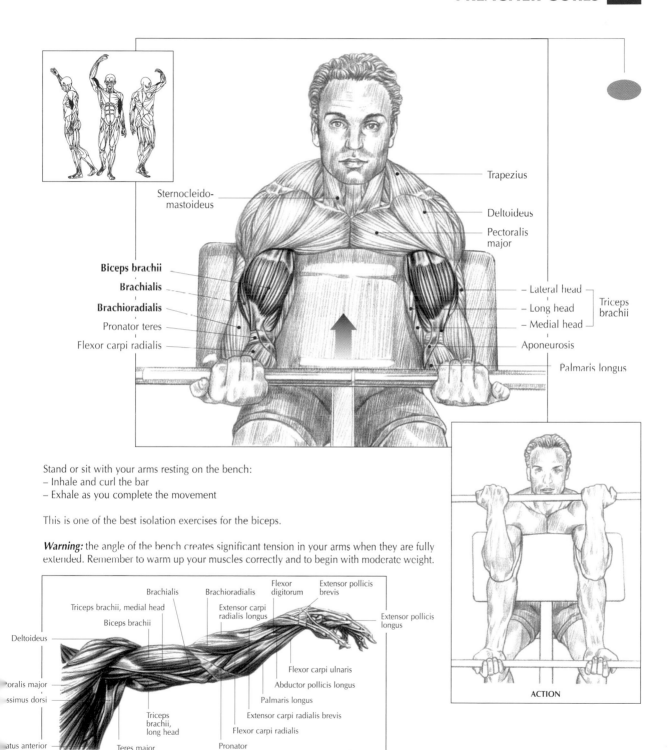

Sternocleido-mastoideus

Trapezius

Deltoideus

Pectoralis major

Biceps brachii

Brachialis

Brachioradialis

Pronator teres

Flexor carpi radialis

– Lateral head

– Long head Triceps brachii

– Medial head

Aponeurosis

Palmaris longus

Stand or sit with your arms resting on the bench:
– Inhale and curl the bar
– Exhale as you complete the movement

This is one of the best isolation exercises for the biceps.

Warning: the angle of the bench creates significant tension in your arms when they are fully extended. Remember to warm up your muscles correctly and to begin with moderate weight.

Triceps brachii, medial head

Brachialis

Biceps brachii

Deltoideus

oralis major

ssimus dorsi

atus anterior

Teres major

Triceps brachii, long head

Brachioradialis

Extensor carpi radialis longus

Flexor digitorum

Extensor pollicis brevis

Extensor pollicis longus

Flexor carpi ulnaris

Abductor pollicis longus

Palmaris longus

Extensor carpi radialis brevis

Flexor carpi radialis

Pronator teres

ACTION

9 REVERSE CURLS

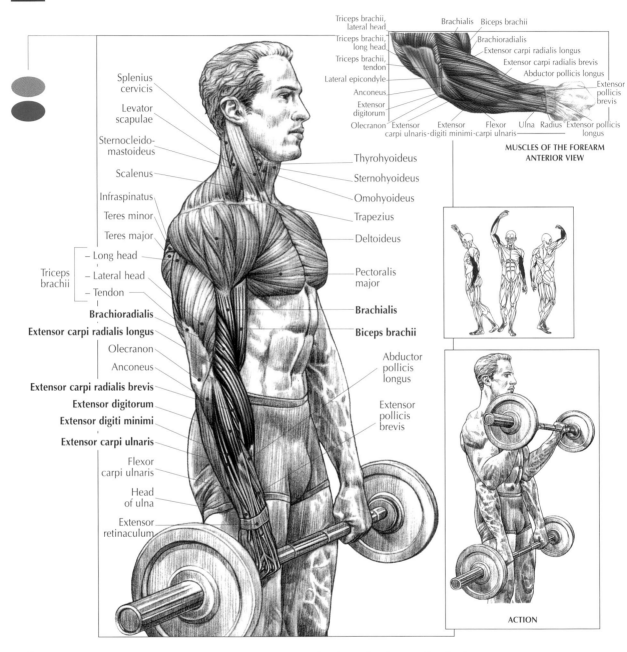

MUSCLES OF THE FOREARM ANTERIOR VIEW

Triceps brachii, lateral head
Triceps brachii, long head
Triceps brachii, tendon
Lateral epicondyle
Anconeus
Extensor digitorum
Olecranon
Extensor carpi ulnaris-digiti minimi-carpi ulnaris
Brachialis
Biceps brachii
Brachioradialis
Extensor carpi radialis longus
Extensor carpi radialis brevis
Abductor pollicis longus
Extensor pollicis brevis
Flexor
Ulna
Radius
Extensor pollicis longus

Splenius cervicis
Levator scapulae
Sternocleido-mastoideus
Scalenus
Infraspinatus
Teres minor
Teres major
Triceps brachii
– Long head
– Lateral head
– Tendon
Brachioradialis
Extensor carpi radialis longus
Olecranon
Anconeus
Extensor carpi radialis brevis
Extensor digitorum
Extensor digiti minimi
Extensor carpi ulnaris
Flexor carpi ulnaris
Head of ulna
Extensor retinaculum

Thyrohyoideus
Sternohyoideus
Omohyoideus
Trapezius
Deltoideus
Pectoralis major
Brachialis
Biceps brachii
Abductor pollicis longus
Extensor pollicis brevis

ACTION

Stand with your feet slightly apart and your arms straight, using an overhand grip (thumbs toward each other):
– Inhale and curl the bar
– Exhale as you complete the movement

This exercise works the extensors of the wrist and fingers. It works the brachioradialis, brachialis, and, to a lesser degree, the biceps.

Note: this is an excellent movement for strengthening the wrist joint. The predominance of the wrist flexors over the wrist extensors often causes imbalance and weakens the wrist. For this reason, this exercise has been integrated into many boxers' training programs. Many bench press champions use it to prevent their wrists from shaking when using heavy weight.

REVERSE WRIST CURLS 10

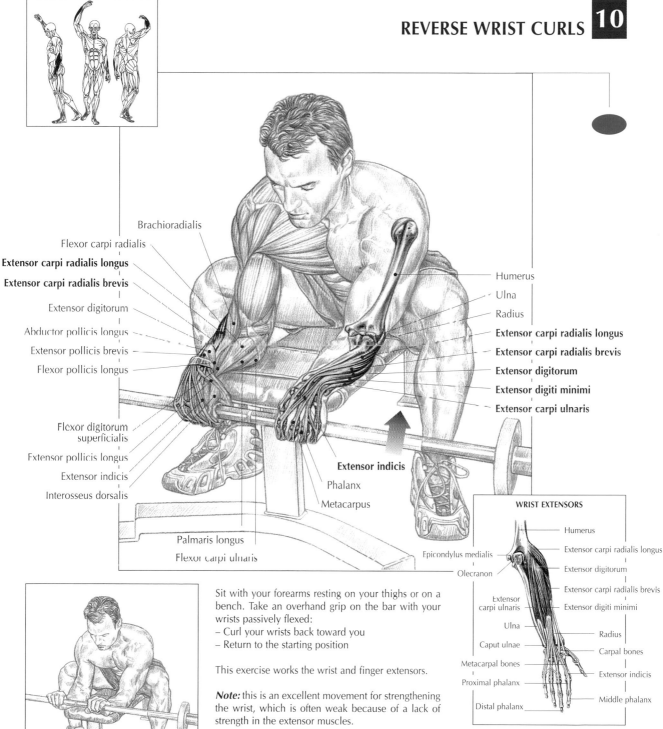

Brachioradialis

Flexor carpi radialis

Extensor carpi radialis longus

Extensor carpi radialis brevis

Extensor digitorum

Abductor pollicis longus

Extensor pollicis brevis

Flexor pollicis longus

Flexor digitorum superficialis

Extensor pollicis longus

Extensor indicis

Interosseus dorsalis

Humerus

Ulna

Radius

Extensor carpi radialis longus

Extensor carpi radialis brevis

Extensor digitorum

Extensor digiti minimi

Extensor carpi ulnaris

Extensor indicis

Phalanx

Metacarpus

Palmaris longus

Flexor carpi ulnaris

WRIST EXTENSORS

Epicondylus medialis

Olecranon

Extensor carpi ulnaris

Ulna

Caput ulnae

Metacarpal bones

Proximal phalanx

Distal phalanx

Humerus

Extensor carpi radialis longus

Extensor digitorum

Extensor carpi radialis brevis

Extensor digiti minimi

Radius

Carpal bones

Extensor indicis

Middle phalanx

Sit with your forearms resting on your thighs or on a bench. Take an overhand grip on the bar with your wrists passively flexed:
– Curl your wrists back toward you
– Return to the starting position

This exercise works the wrist and finger extensors.

Note: this is an excellent movement for strengthening the wrist, which is often weak because of a lack of strength in the extensor muscles.

END OF MOVEMENT

11 WRIST CURLS

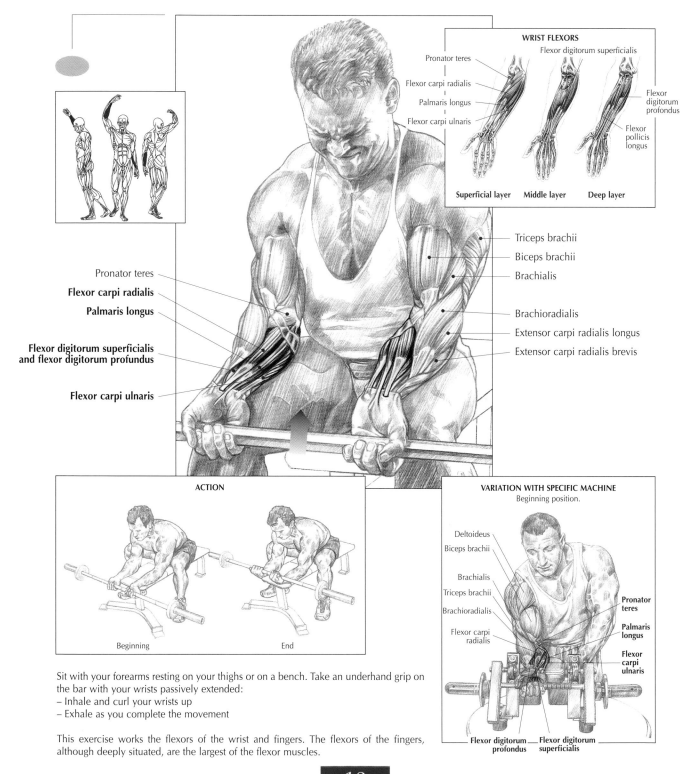

WRIST FLEXORS

Pronator teres

Flexor carpi radialis

Palmaris longus

Flexor carpi ulnaris

Flexor digitorum superficialis

Flexor digitorum profondus

Flexor pollicis longus

Superficial layer — **Middle layer** — **Deep layer**

Triceps brachii

Biceps brachii

Brachialis

Brachioradialis

Extensor carpi radialis longus

Extensor carpi radialis brevis

Pronator teres

Flexor carpi radialis

Palmaris longus

Flexor digitorum superficialis and flexor digitorum profundus

Flexor carpi ulnaris

ACTION

Beginning — End

VARIATION WITH SPECIFIC MACHINE
Beginning position.

Deltoideus

Biceps brachii

Brachialis

Triceps brachii

Brachioradialis

Flexor carpi radialis

Pronator teres

Palmaris longus

Flexor carpi ulnaris

Flexor digitorum profondus — **Flexor digitorum superficialis**

Sit with your forearms resting on your thighs or on a bench. Take an underhand grip on the bar with your wrists passively extended:
– Inhale and curl your wrists up
– Exhale as you complete the movement

This exercise works the flexors of the wrist and fingers. The flexors of the fingers, although deeply situated, are the largest of the flexor muscles.

PUSHDOWNS 12

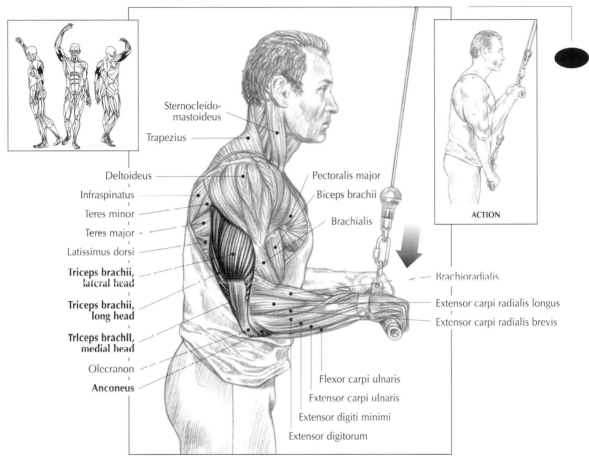

Sternocleido-mastoideus

Trapezius

Deltoideus

Infraspinatus

Teres minor

Teres major

Latissimus dorsi

Triceps brachii, lateral head

Triceps brachii, long head

Triceps brachii, medial head

Olecranon

Anconeus

Pectoralis major

Biceps brachii

Brachialis

Brachioradialis

Extensor carpi radialis longus

Extensor carpi radialis brevis

Flexor carpi ulnaris

Extensor carpi ulnaris

Extensor digiti minimi

Extensor digitorum

ACTION

Stand facing the machine with your hands on the bar and your elbows against your sides:
– Inhale and straighten your arms, but don't separate your elbows from your sides
– Exhale as you complete the movement

This isolation exercise works the triceps and the anconeus.

You can perform an effective variation of this movement with a rope instead of the bar to work the lateral head of the triceps more intensely. Use an underhand grip to place emphasis on the medial head of the triceps.

At the end of the movement, hold an isometric contraction for one or two seconds to feel the effort more intensely.

If you use a heavy weight, lean slightly forward at the waist for more stability.

This exercise is very easy to perform and can be done by beginners to help develop strength before moving to more difficult exercises.

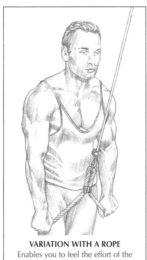

VARIATION WITH A ROPE
Enables you to feel the effort of the lateral head of the triceps more intensely.

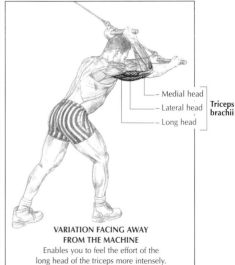

Medial head

Lateral head

Long head

Triceps brachii

VARIATION FACING AWAY FROM THE MACHINE
Enables you to feel the effort of the long head of the triceps more intensely.

13 REVERSE PUSHDOWNS

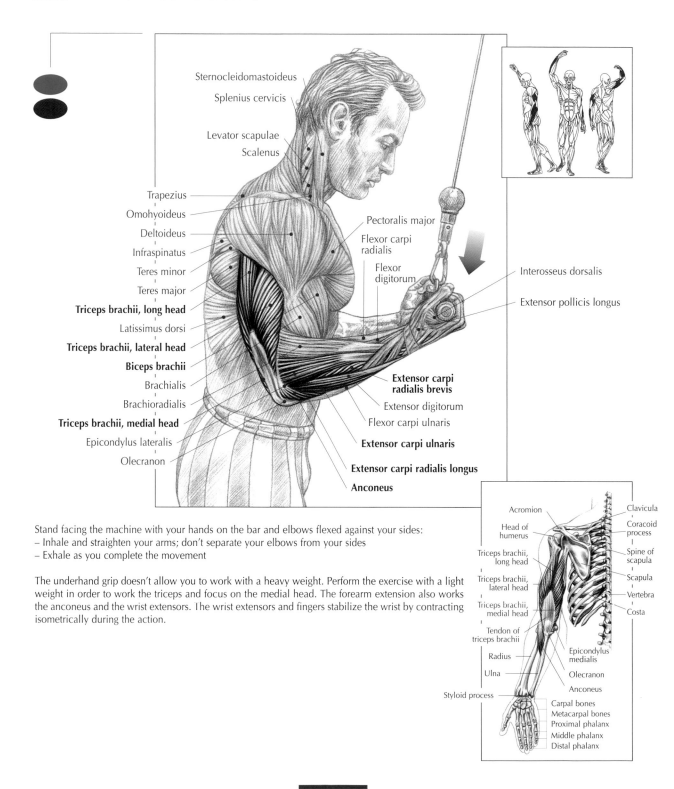

Sternocleidomastoideus

Splenius cervicis

Levator scapulae

Scalenus

Trapezius

Omohyoideus

Deltoideus

Infraspinatus

Teres minor

Teres major

Triceps brachii, long head

Latissimus dorsi

Triceps brachii, lateral head

Biceps brachii

Brachialis

Brachioradialis

Triceps brachii, medial head

Epicondylus lateralis

Olecranon

Pectoralis major

Flexor carpi radialis

Flexor digitorum

Interosseus dorsalis

Extensor pollicis longus

Extensor carpi radialis brevis

Extensor digitorum

Flexor carpi ulnaris

Extensor carpi ulnaris

Extensor carpi radialis longus

Anconeus

Acromion

Head of humerus

Triceps brachii, long head

Triceps brachii, lateral head

Triceps brachii, medial head

Tendon of triceps brachii

Radius

Ulna

Styloid process

Clavicula

Coracoid process

Spine of scapula

Scapula

Vertebra

Costa

Epicondylus medialis

Olecranon

Anconeus

Carpal bones
Metacarpal bones
Proximal phalanx
Middle phalanx
Distal phalanx

Stand facing the machine with your hands on the bar and elbows flexed against your sides:
– Inhale and straighten your arms; don't separate your elbows from your sides
– Exhale as you complete the movement

The underhand grip doesn't allow you to work with a heavy weight. Perform the exercise with a light weight in order to work the triceps and focus on the medial head. The forearm extension also works the anconeus and the wrist extensors. The wrist extensors and fingers stabilize the wrist by contracting isometrically during the action.

ONE-ARM REVERSE PUSHDOWNS 14

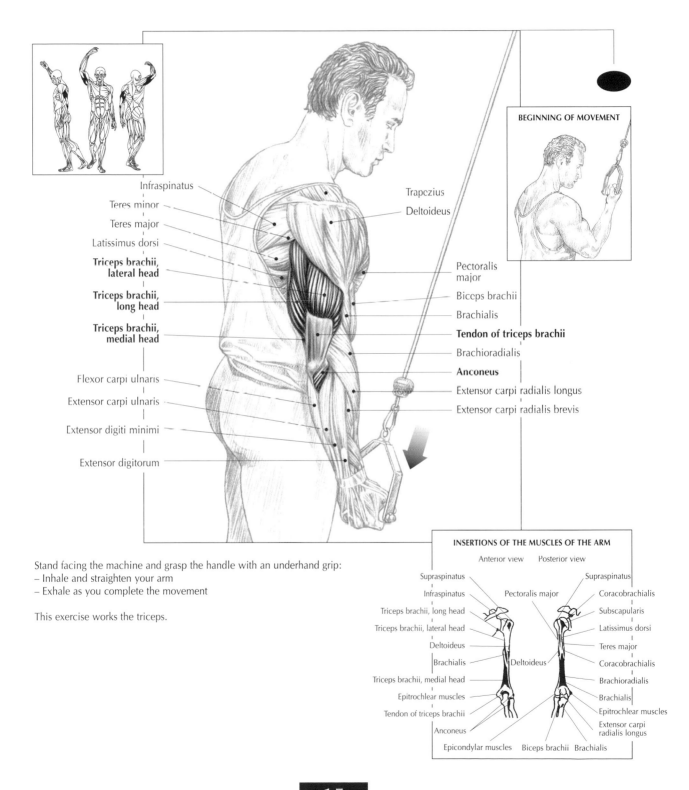

BEGINNING OF MOVEMENT

Infraspinatus

Teres minor

Teres major

Latissimus dorsi

Triceps brachii, lateral head

Triceps brachii, long head

Triceps brachii, medial head

Flexor carpi ulnaris

Extensor carpi ulnaris

Extensor digiti minimi

Extensor digitorum

Trapezius

Deltoideus

Pectoralis major

Biceps brachii

Brachialis

Tendon of triceps brachii

Brachioradialis

Anconeus

Extensor carpi radialis longus

Extensor carpi radialis brevis

Stand facing the machine and grasp the handle with an underhand grip:
– Inhale and straighten your arm
– Exhale as you complete the movement

This exercise works the triceps.

INSERTIONS OF THE MUSCLES OF THE ARM

Anterior view   Posterior view

Supraspinatus

Infraspinatus

Triceps brachii, long head

Triceps brachii, lateral head

Deltoideus

Brachialis

Triceps brachii, medial head

Epitrochlear muscles

Tendon of triceps brachii

Anconeus

Epicondylar muscles

Pectoralis major

Deltoideus

Biceps brachii   Brachialis

Supraspinatus

Coracobrachialis

Subscapularis

Latissimus dorsi

Teres major

Coracobrachialis

Brachioradialis

Brachialis

Epitrochlear muscles

Extensor carpi radialis longus

15 TRICEPS EXTENSIONS

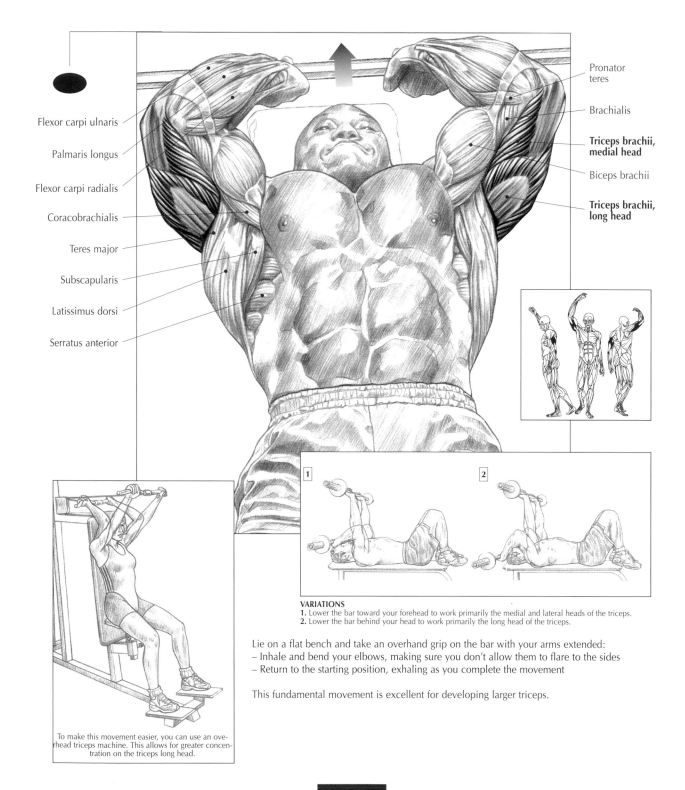

Flexor carpi ulnaris

Palmaris longus

Flexor carpi radialis

Coracobrachialis

Teres major

Subscapularis

Latissimus dorsi

Serratus anterior

Pronator teres

Brachialis

Triceps brachii, medial head

Biceps brachii

Triceps brachii, long head

To make this movement easier, you can use an overhead triceps machine. This allows for greater concentration on the triceps long head.

VARIATIONS
1. Lower the bar toward your forehead to work primarily the medial and lateral heads of the triceps.
2. Lower the bar behind your head to work primarily the long head of the triceps.

Lie on a flat bench and take an overhand grip on the bar with your arms extended:
– Inhale and bend your elbows, making sure you don't allow them to flare to the sides
– Return to the starting position, exhaling as you complete the movement

This fundamental movement is excellent for developing larger triceps.

DUMBBELL TRICEPS EXTENSIONS **16**

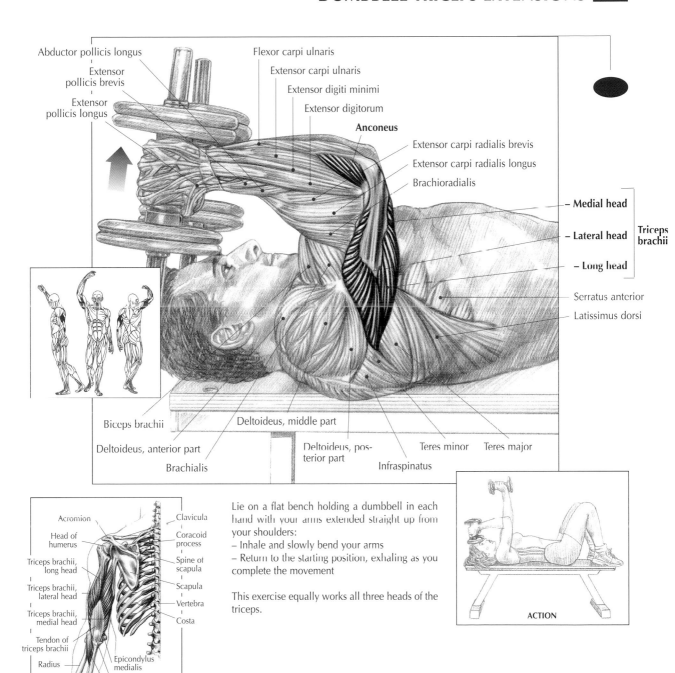

Abductor pollicis longus
Extensor pollicis brevis
Extensor pollicis longus

Flexor carpi ulnaris
Extensor carpi ulnaris
Extensor digiti minimi
Extensor digitorum
Anconeus
Extensor carpi radialis brevis
Extensor carpi radialis longus
Brachioradialis

– **Medial head**
– **Lateral head**   **Triceps brachii**
– **Long head**

Serratus anterior
Latissimus dorsi

Biceps brachii
Deltoideus, anterior part
Brachialis
Deltoideus, middle part
Deltoideus, posterior part
Infraspinatus
Teres minor
Teres major

Acromion
Head of humerus
Triceps brachii, long head
Triceps brachii, lateral head
Triceps brachii, medial head
Tendon of triceps brachii
Radius
Ulna
Styloid process
Clavicula
Coracoid process
Spine of scapula
Scapula
Vertebra
Costa
Epicondylus medialis
Olecranon
Anconeus
Carpal bones
Metacarpal bones
Proximal phalanx
Middle phalanx
Distal phalanx

Lie on a flat bench holding a dumbbell in each hand with your arms extended straight up from your shoulders:
– Inhale and slowly bend your arms
– Return to the starting position, exhaling as you complete the movement

This exercise equally works all three heads of the triceps.

ACTION

17 ONE-ARM DUMBBELL TRICEPS EXTENSIONS

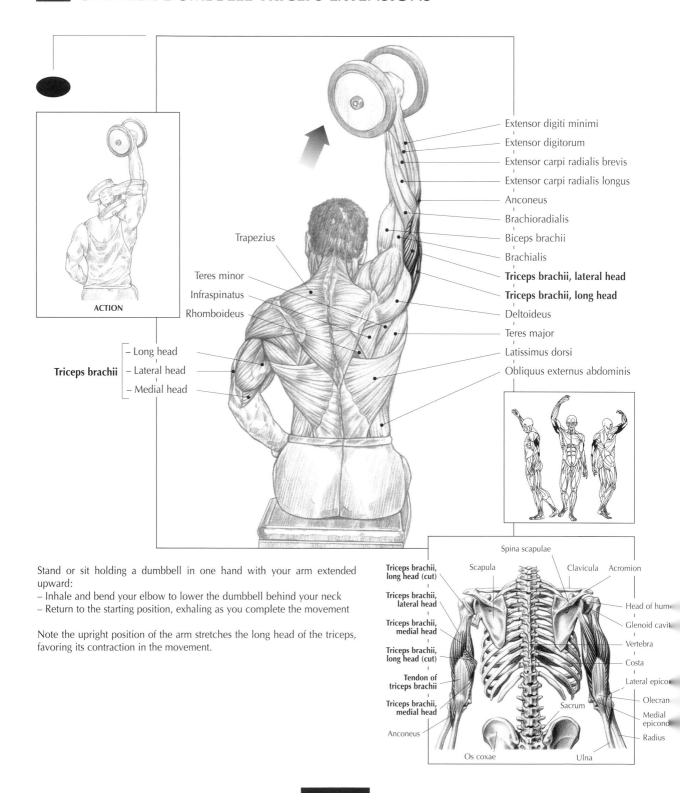

ACTION

Trapezius

Teres minor

Infraspinatus

Rhomboideus

Triceps brachii
– Long head
– Lateral head
– Medial head

Extensor digiti minimi

Extensor digitorum

Extensor carpi radialis brevis

Extensor carpi radialis longus

Anconeus

Brachioradialis

Biceps brachii

Brachialis

Triceps brachii, lateral head

Triceps brachii, long head

Deltoideus

Teres major

Latissimus dorsi

Obliquus externus abdominis

Spina scapulae

Scapula

Clavicula   Acromion

Triceps brachii, long head (cut)

Triceps brachii, lateral head

Triceps brachii, medial head

Triceps brachii, long head (cut)

Tendon of triceps brachii

Triceps brachii, medial head

Anconeus

Head of hume

Glenoid cavit

Vertebra

Costa

Lateral epico

Olecran

Medial epicond

Radius

Sacrum

Os coxae

Ulna

Stand or sit holding a dumbbell in one hand with your arm extended upward:
– Inhale and bend your elbow to lower the dumbbell behind your neck
– Return to the starting position, exhaling as you complete the movement

Note the upright position of the arm stretches the long head of the triceps, favoring its contraction in the movement.

SEATED DUMBBELL TRICEPS EXTENSIONS 18

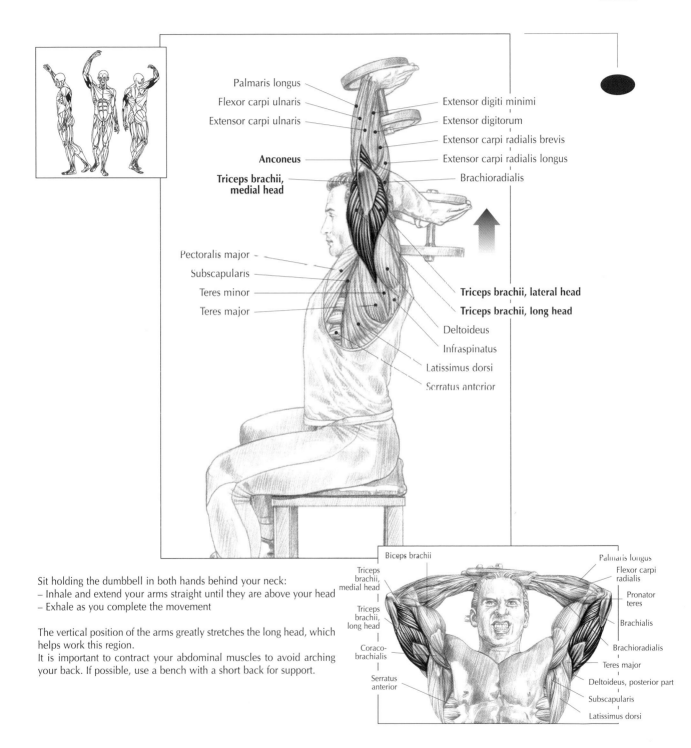

Palmaris longus
Flexor carpi ulnaris
Extensor carpi ulnaris
Anconeus
Triceps brachii, medial head

Extensor digiti minimi
Extensor digitorum
Extensor carpi radialis brevis
Extensor carpi radialis longus
Brachioradialis

Pectoralis major
Subscapularis
Teres minor
Teres major

Triceps brachii, lateral head
Triceps brachii, long head
Deltoideus
Infraspinatus
Latissimus dorsi
Serratus anterior

Biceps brachii
Triceps brachii, medial head
Triceps brachii, long head
Coraco-brachialis
Serratus anterior

Palmaris longus
Flexor carpi radialis
Pronator teres
Brachialis
Brachioradialis
Teres major
Deltoideus, posterior part
Subscapularis
Latissimus dorsi

Sit holding the dumbbell in both hands behind your neck:
– Inhale and extend your arms straight until they are above your head
– Exhale as you complete the movement

The vertical position of the arms greatly stretches the long head, which helps work this region.
It is important to contract your abdominal muscles to avoid arching your back. If possible, use a bench with a short back for support.

19 SEATED EZ-BAR TRICEPS EXTENSIONS

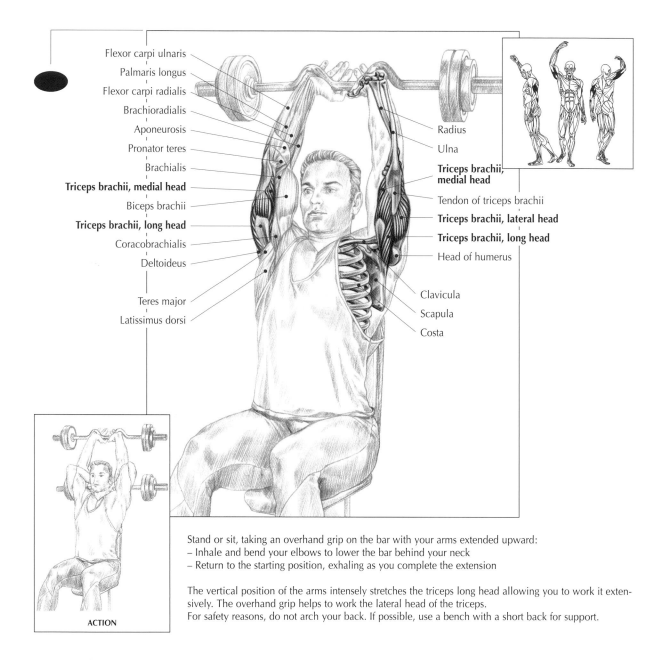

Flexor carpi ulnaris
Palmaris longus
Flexor carpi radialis
Brachioradialis
Aponeurosis
Pronator teres
Brachialis
Triceps brachii, medial head
Biceps brachii
Triceps brachii, long head
Coracobrachialis
Deltoideus
Teres major
Latissimus dorsi

Radius
Ulna
Triceps brachii, medial head
Tendon of triceps brachii
Triceps brachii, lateral head
Triceps brachii, long head
Head of humerus
Clavicula
Scapula
Costa

ACTION

Stand or sit, taking an overhand grip on the bar with your arms extended upward:
– Inhale and bend your elbows to lower the bar behind your neck
– Return to the starting position, exhaling as you complete the extension

The vertical position of the arms intensely stretches the triceps long head allowing you to work it extensively. The overhand grip helps to work the lateral head of the triceps.
For safety reasons, do not arch your back. If possible, use a bench with a short back for support.

TRICEPS KICKBACKS 20

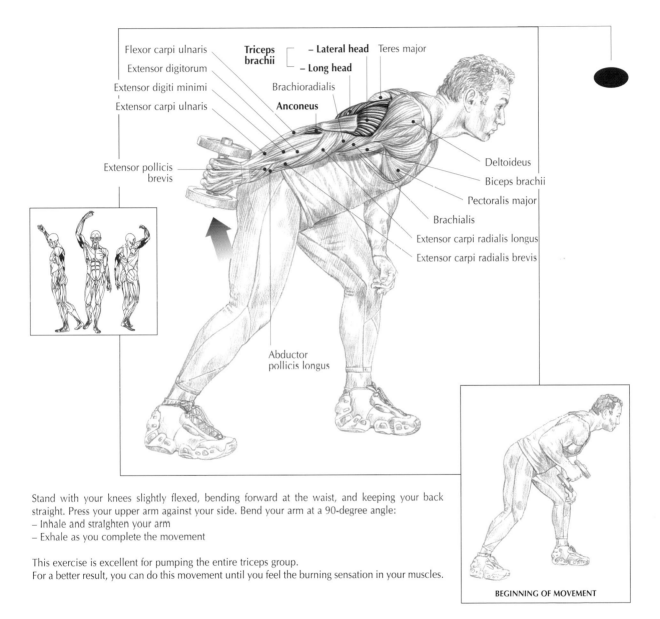

Flexor carpi ulnaris
Extensor digitorum
Extensor digiti minimi
Extensor carpi ulnaris
Extensor pollicis brevis
Abductor pollicis longus

Triceps brachii
– Lateral head
– Long head
Brachioradialis
Anconeus

Teres major
Deltoideus
Biceps brachii
Pectoralis major
Brachialis
Extensor carpi radialis longus
Extensor carpi radialis brevis

BEGINNING OF MOVEMENT

Stand with your knees slightly flexed, bending forward at the waist, and keeping your back straight. Press your upper arm against your side. Bend your arm at a 90-degree angle:
– Inhale and straighten your arm
– Exhale as you complete the movement

This exercise is excellent for pumping the entire triceps group.
For a better result, you can do this movement until you feel the burning sensation in your muscles.

21 TRICEPS DIPS

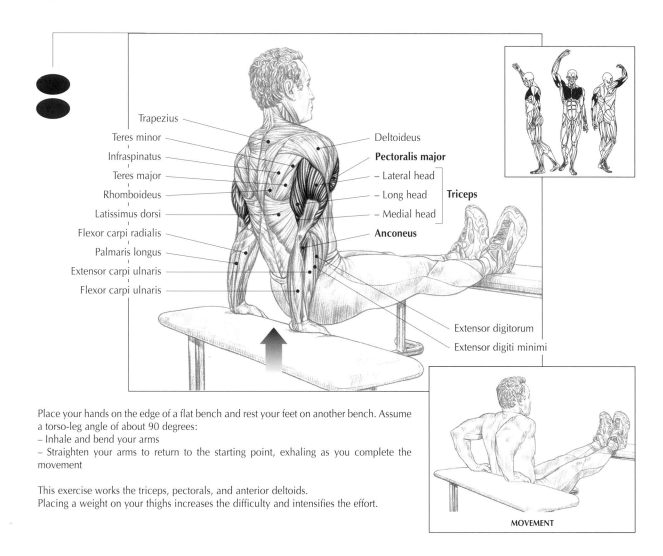

Trapezius
Teres minor
Infraspinatus
Teres major
Rhomboideus
Latissimus dorsi
Flexor carpi radialis
Palmaris longus
Extensor carpi ulnaris
Flexor carpi ulnaris

Deltoideus
Pectoralis major
– Lateral head
– Long head   **Triceps**
– Medial head
Anconeus

Extensor digitorum
Extensor digiti minimi

MOVEMENT

Place your hands on the edge of a flat bench and rest your feet on another bench. Assume a torso-leg angle of about 90 degrees:
– Inhale and bend your arms
– Straighten your arms to return to the starting point, exhaling as you complete the movement

This exercise works the triceps, pectorals, and anterior deltoids.
Placing a weight on your thighs increases the difficulty and intensifies the effort.

2 SHOULDERS

1. Back Press
2. Front Press
3. Dumbbell Press
4. One-Arm Dumbbell Press
5. Lateral Raises
6. Bent-Over Lateral Raises
7. Front Raises
8. Side-Lying Lateral Raises
9. Low Pulley Lateral Raises
10. Low Pulley Front Raises
11. Low Pulley Bent-Over Lateral Raises
12. One-Dumbbell Front Raises
13. Barbell Front Raises
14. Upright Rows
15. Nautilus Lateral Raises
16. Pec Deck Rear Delt Laterals

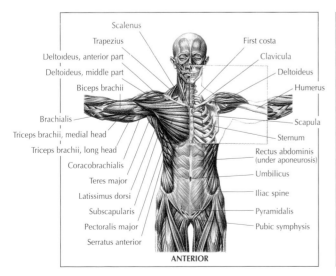

ANTERIOR

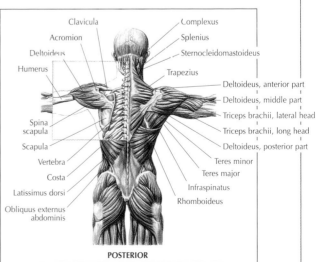

POSTERIOR

1 BACK PRESS

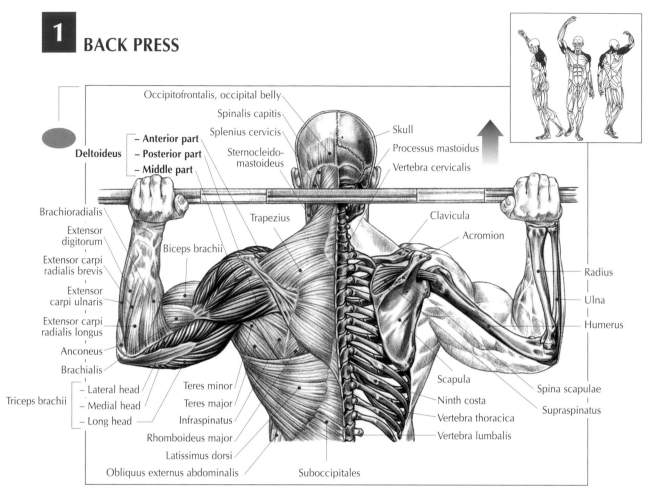

Occipitofrontalis, occipital belly
Spinalis capitis
Splenius cervicis
Sternocleido-mastoideus

Deltoideus
– **Anterior part**
– **Posterior part**
– **Middle part**

Skull
Processus mastoidus
Vertebra cervicalis

Brachioradialis
Extensor digitorum
Extensor carpi radialis brevis
Extensor carpi ulnaris
Extensor carpi radialis longus
Anconeus
Brachialis

Biceps brachii
Trapezius

Clavicula
Acromion

Radius
Ulna
Humerus

Triceps brachii
– Lateral head
– Medial head
– Long head

Teres minor
Teres major
Infraspinatus
Rhomboideus major
Latissimus dorsi
Obliquus externus abdominalis

Scapula
Ninth costa
Vertebra thoracica
Vertebra lumbalis
Suboccipitales

Spina scapulae
Supraspinatus

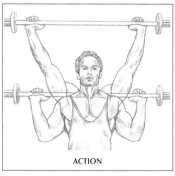

ACTION

Sit on a bench with your back straight. Grasp a barbell with an overhand grip and rest the barbell across your shoulders behind your neck:
– Inhale and press the barbell directly above your head without arching your back
– Exhale as you complete the movement

This exercise works the deltoids, particularly the medial part, and the upper trapezius, triceps, and serratus anterior. It also works the rhomboids, infraspinatus, teres minor, and supraspinatus.
You can also perform this movement while standing or by setting the bar on a rack. There are many machines that allow you to do this exercise with less concentration on form and safety.

Note: to avoid traumatizing the shoulder joint, which is particularly delicate, rest the bar higher or lower behind your neck according to your body type and flexibility. This exercise can be strenuous on the rotator cuff muscles and should be performed with caution.

FRONT PRESS **2**

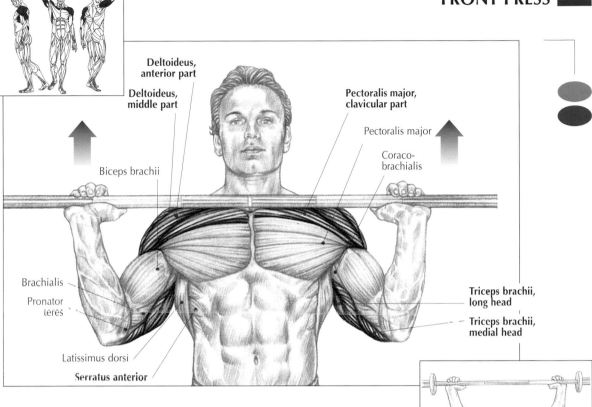

Deltoideus, anterior part

Deltoideus, middle part

Pectoralis major, clavicular part

Pectoralis major

Coraco-brachialis

Biceps brachii

Brachialis

Pronator teres

Latissimus dorsi

Serratus anterior

Triceps brachii, long head

Triceps brachii, medial head

ACTION

Sit with your back straight. Take an overhand grip on the barbell and rest it on your upper chest:
– Inhale and press the barbell straight up
– Exhale at the top of the movement

This basic exercise works the following muscles:
– Anterior and medial deltoids
– Upper pectorals
– Upper trapezius
– Triceps
– Serratus anterior
You can perform this exercise while standing, but you must avoid hyperextension of the spine. Place your elbows slighty forward for more work on the anterior deltoids. To involve the medial deltoids more intensely, flare out your elbows. Many machines and racks allow you to perform this movement with less concentration on the correct position, which helps you focus on the deltoids.

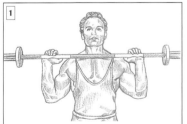

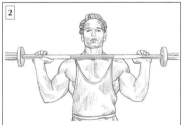

VARIATIONS:
1. *Narrow grip, elbows forward:* primarily works the anterior deltoids and upper pectorals.
2. *Wide grip, elbows flared out:* Primarily works the anterior and medial deltoids.

3 DUMBBELL PRESS

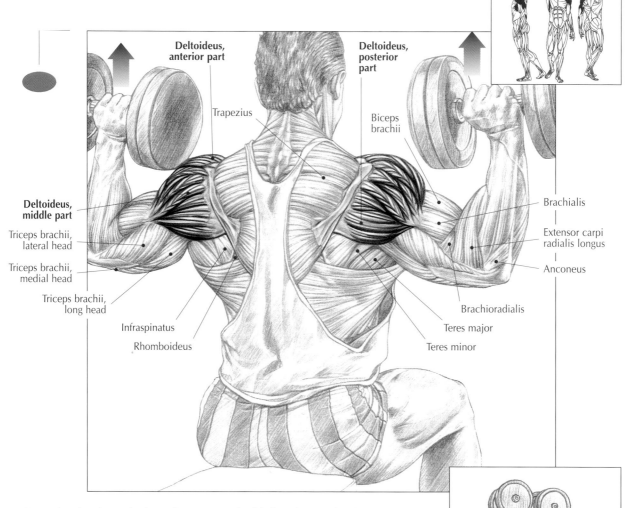

Deltoideus, anterior part

Deltoideus, posterior part

Trapezius

Biceps brachii

Deltoideus, middle part

Triceps brachii, lateral head

Triceps brachii, medial head

Triceps brachii, long head

Infraspinatus

Rhomboideus

Brachialis

Extensor carpi radialis longus

Anconeus

Brachioradialis

Teres major

Teres minor

Sit on a bench with your back straight. Grasp two dumbbells with an overhand grip and lift them to your shoulders, palms facing forward:
– Inhale and press your arms to an extended vertical position
– Exhale as you complete the movement

This exercise uses the deltoids, particularly the medial deltoids, and the upper trapezius, serratus anterior, and triceps.
This movement can also be executed standing and/or with alternating arms. However, the seated version is often used to prevent hyperextension of the spine.

VARIATION
Palms facing toward each other.

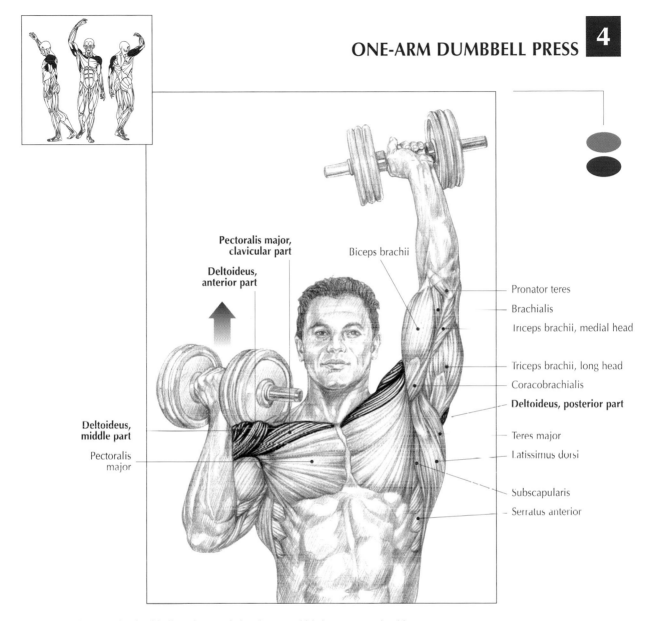

ONE-ARM DUMBBELL PRESS 4

Pectoralis major, clavicular part

Biceps brachii

Deltoideus, anterior part

Pronator teres

Brachialis

Triceps brachii, medial head

Triceps brachii, long head

Coracobrachialis

Deltoideus, posterior part

Teres major

Latissimus dorsi

Subscapularis

Serratus anterior

Deltoideus, middle part

Pectoralis major

Sit on a bench, grasp the dumbbells with an underhand grip, and lift them to your shoulders:
– Inhale and alternately press your arms to an extended vertical position, rotating your wrist so your palm faces forward
– exhale as you complete the movement

This exercise focuses on the deltoids, particularly the anterior deltoids, and the upper pectorals, upper trapezius, serratus anterior, and triceps. You can also do this movement
– sitting against the back of a seat to avoid extreme hyperextension of the spine,
– standing erect, or
– pressing the dumbbells simultaneously.

5 LATERAL RAISES

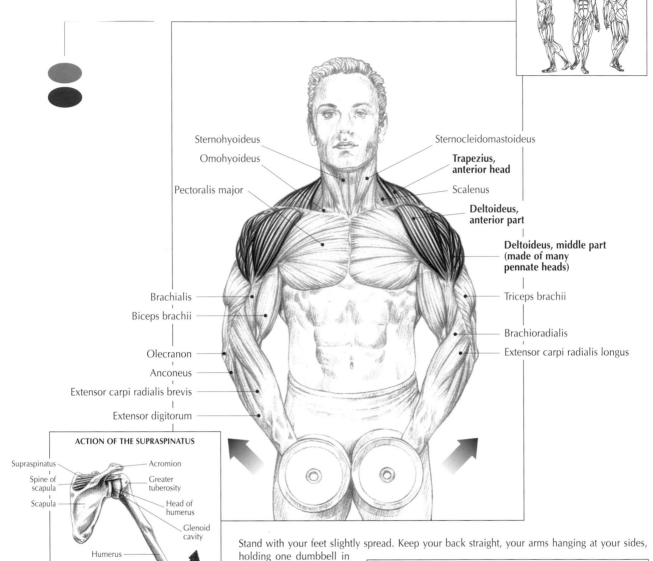

Sternohyoideus

Omohyoideus

Pectoralis major

Sternocleidomastoideus

Trapezius, anterior head

Scalenus

Deltoideus, anterior part

Deltoideus, middle part (made of many pennate heads)

Brachialis

Biceps brachii

Olecranon

Anconeus

Extensor carpi radialis brevis

Extensor digitorum

Triceps brachii

Brachioradialis

Extensor carpi radialis longus

ACTION OF THE SUPRASPINATUS

Supraspinatus

Spine of scapula

Scapula

Acromion

Greater tuberosity

Head of humerus

Glenoid cavity

Humerus

The supraspinatus works with the deltoid to help raise the arm laterally and hold the humerus in place within the joint of the shoulder.

Stand with your feet slightly spread. Keep your back straight, your arms hanging at your sides, holding one dumbbell in each hand:
– Raise the dumbbells to shoulder level, keeping your elbows slightly bent
– Return to the starting position

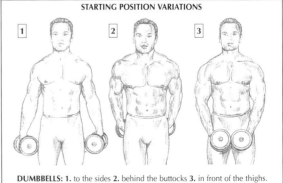

STARTING POSITION VARIATIONS

1 2 3

DUMBBELLS: 1. to the sides **2.** behind the buttocks **3.** in front of the thighs.

This exercise isolates, almost exclusively, the medial deltoids, which are composed of several pennate heads converging on the humerus. They are involved when you hold relatively heavy weight and enable you to move your arms with precision in every plane. It is more effective to train this muscle by starting at different positions (hands to the sides, behind the buttocks, or in front of the thighs) to involve the medial deltoids completely.

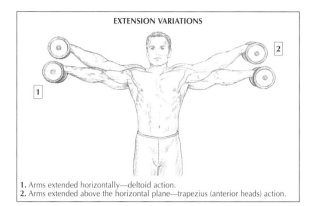

EXTENSION VARIATIONS

1. Arms extended horizontally—deltoid action.
2. Arms extended above the horizontal plane—trapezius (anterior heads) action.

This exercise also works the supraspinatus, located beneath the deltoid muscle in the supraspinatus fossa of the scapula and inserted into the humeral large tuberosity.

Because body types vary, you must find an optimal angle of work that meets the needs of your physique.

You can stress the upper part of the trapezius by raising the arms above the horizontal plane. However, many bodybuilders avoid doing this to place primary emphasis on the medial deltoid.

This exercise is never performed with heavy weight. Sets of 10 to 25 reps give the best results if you vary the angle of work, spend little time recovering, and train to the point of feeling the burning sensation.

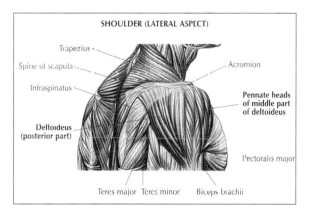

SHOULDER (LATERAL ASPECT)

- Trapezius
- Spine of scapula
- Infraspinatus
- Deltoideus (posterior part)
- Acromion
- Pennate heads of middle part of deltoideus
- Pectoralis major
- Teres major
- Teres minor
- Biceps brachii

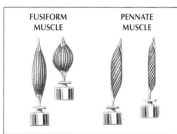

FUSIFORM MUSCLE — **PENNATE MUSCLE**

A pennate muscle proportionately moves heavier loads than a fusiform muscle, but for shorter distances. When performing lateral raises, the pennate heads of the medial deltoid—very powerful, but with a weak contraction potential—work synergistically with the anterior and posterior heads of the deltoid to bring the arm horizontal.

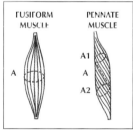

FUSIFORM MUSCLE — **PENNATE MUSCLE**

A
A1
A
A2

The amount of actin* and myosin* filaments of a fusiform muscle is equal to its crosssection (A).

The amount of actin and myosin filaments of a pennate muscle equals the (A) amount of the A1 and A2 oblique sections.

*Muscle motor elements whose maximal contraction force is equal to about 5 kg/cm² of section.

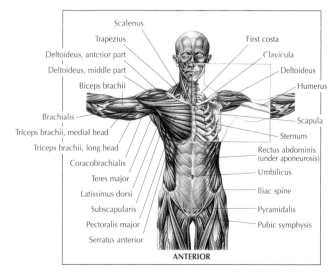

- Scalenus
- Trapezius
- Deltoideus, anterior part
- Deltoideus, middle part
- Biceps brachii
- Brachialis
- Triceps brachii, medial head
- Triceps brachii, long head
- Coracobrachialis
- Teres major
- Latissimus dorsi
- Subscapularis
- Pectoralis major
- Serratus anterior
- First costa
- Clavicula
- Deltoideus
- Humerus
- Scapula
- Sternum
- Rectus abdominis (under aponeurosis)
- Umbilicus
- Iliac spine
- Pyramidalis
- Pubic symphysis

ANTERIOR

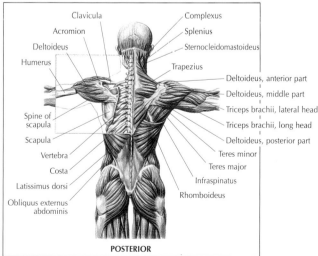

- Clavicula
- Acromion
- Deltoideus
- Humerus
- Spine of scapula
- Scapula
- Vertebra
- Costa
- Latissimus dorsi
- Obliquus externus abdominis
- Complexus
- Splenius
- Sternocleidomastoideus
- Trapezius
- Deltoideus, anterior part
- Deltoideus, middle part
- Triceps brachii, lateral head
- Triceps brachii, long head
- Deltoideus, posterior part
- Teres minor
- Teres major
- Infraspinatus
- Rhomboideus

POSTERIOR

6 BENT-OVER LATERAL RAISES

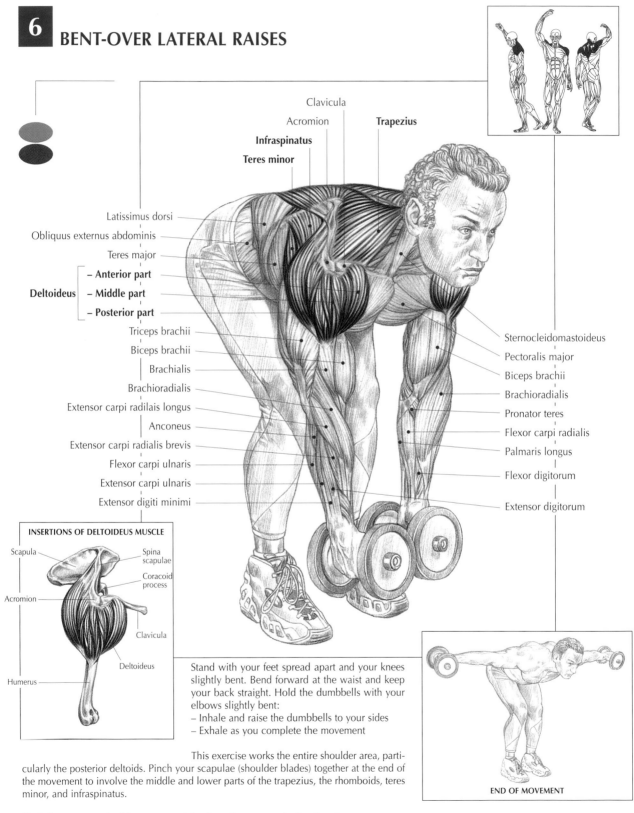

Clavicula

Acromion

Infraspinatus

Teres minor

Trapezius

Latissimus dorsi

Obliquus externus abdominis

Teres major

Deltoideus
- **Anterior part**
- **Middle part**
- **Posterior part**

Triceps brachii

Biceps brachii

Brachialis

Brachioradialis

Extensor carpi radilais longus

Anconeus

Extensor carpi radialis brevis

Flexor carpi ulnaris

Extensor carpi ulnaris

Extensor digiti minimi

Sternocleidomastoideus

Pectoralis major

Biceps brachii

Brachioradialis

Pronator teres

Flexor carpi radialis

Palmaris longus

Flexor digitorum

Extensor digitorum

INSERTIONS OF DELTOIDEUS MUSCLE

Scapula

Spina scapulae

Coracoid process

Acromion

Clavicula

Deltoideus

Humerus

Stand with your feet spread apart and your knees slightly bent. Bend forward at the waist and keep your back straight. Hold the dumbbells with your elbows slightly bent:
- Inhale and raise the dumbbells to your sides
- Exhale as you complete the movement

This exercise works the entire shoulder area, particularly the posterior deltoids. Pinch your scapulae (shoulder blades) together at the end of the movement to involve the middle and lower parts of the trapezius, the rhomboids, teres minor, and infraspinatus.

END OF MOVEMENT

Variation: you can do this movement lying face down on an incline bench.

FRONT RAISES 7

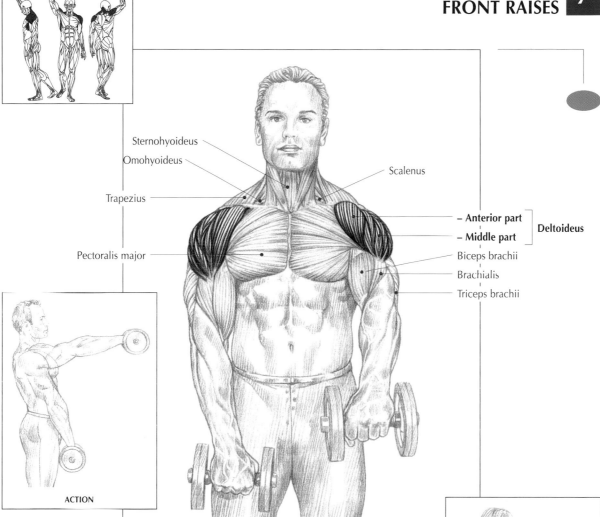

Sternohyoideus
Omohyoideus
Trapezius
Pectoralis major

Scalenus

– Anterior part
– Middle part Deltoideus

Biceps brachii
Brachialis
Triceps brachii

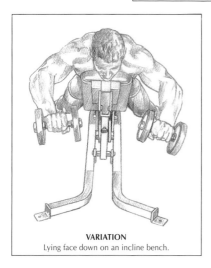

ACTION

Stand with your feet slightly apart. Hold the dumbbells with your palms down (overhand grip), resting the dumbbells on your thighs or slightly to your sides:
– Inhale and alternate sides, raising the dumbbells forward to shoulder height
– Exhale as you complete the movement

This exercise places primary emphasis on the anterior deltoids and upper pectorals and, to a lesser extent, on the middle deltoids. Every arm raise exercise also involves the muscles that attach the scapulae (shoulder blades) to the rib cage, such as the serratus anterior and rhomboids (which stabilize the humerus in its movements).

VARIATION
Lying face down on an incline bench.

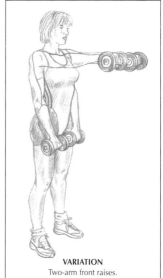

VARIATION
Two-arm front raises.

8 SIDE-LYING LATERAL RAISES

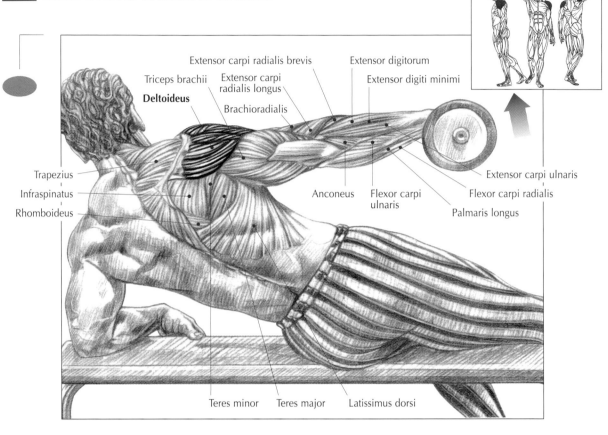

Extensor carpi radialis brevis
Triceps brachii
Extensor carpi radialis longus
Deltoideus
Brachioradialis
Extensor digitorum
Extensor digiti minimi
Trapezius
Infraspinatus
Rhomboideus
Anconeus
Flexor carpi ulnaris
Extensor carpi ulnaris
Flexor carpi radialis
Palmaris longus
Teres minor
Teres major
Latissimus dorsi

Lie on your side on the floor or a bench, holding a dumbbell with an overhand grip:
– Inhale and raise your arm
– Exhale as you complete the movement

Unlike standing raises, which gradually work the muscle to maximum intensity at the end of the movement (when you bring your arms to a horizontal position), this exercise involves the deltoids differently, concentrating the effort at the beginning of the movement.

Note: this movement emphasizes the supraspinatus, mainly working at the beginning of the movement. Vary the starting position (dumbbell placed forward, on the thigh, or toward the rear) to place the emphasis on all of the deltoid heads.

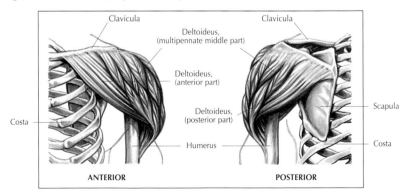

Clavicula
Deltoideus, (multipennate middle part)
Deltoideus, (anterior part)
Clavicula
Costa
Deltoideus, (posterior part)
Scapula
Humerus
Costa

ANTERIOR   **POSTERIOR**

LOW PULLEY LATERAL RAISES 9

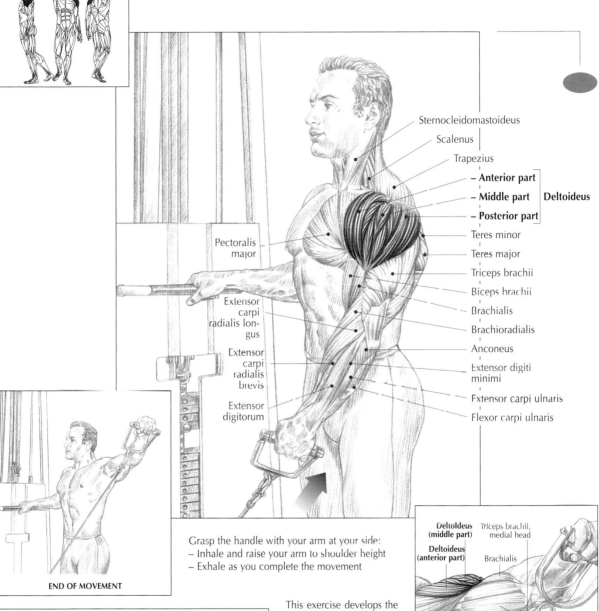

Sternocleidomastoideus

Scalenus

Trapezius

– **Anterior part**
– **Middle part**   Deltoideus
– **Posterior part**

Teres minor

Teres major

Triceps brachii

Biceps brachii

Brachialis

Brachioradialis

Anconeus

Extensor digiti minimi

Extensor carpi ulnaris

Flexor carpi ulnaris

Pectoralis major

Extensor carpi radialis longus

Extensor carpi radialis brevis

Extensor digitorum

Deltoideus (middle part)   Triceps brachii, medial head

Deltoideus (anterior part)   Brachialis

Biceps brachii

Triceps brachii, long head

Coracobrachialis

Teres major

Latissimus dorsi

END OF MOVEMENT

Grasp the handle with your arm at your side:
– Inhale and raise your arm to shoulder height
– Exhale as you complete the movement

This exercise develops the deltoid, particularly the multipenniform medial head. You should vary the angle of work to stress all the deltoid parts.

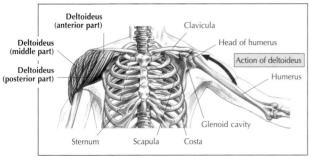

Deltoideus (anterior part)

Clavicula

Deltoideus (middle part)

Head of humerus

Action of deltoideus

Deltoideus (posterior part)

Humerus

Glenoid cavity

Sternum   Scapula   Costa

10 LOW PULLEY FRONT RAISES

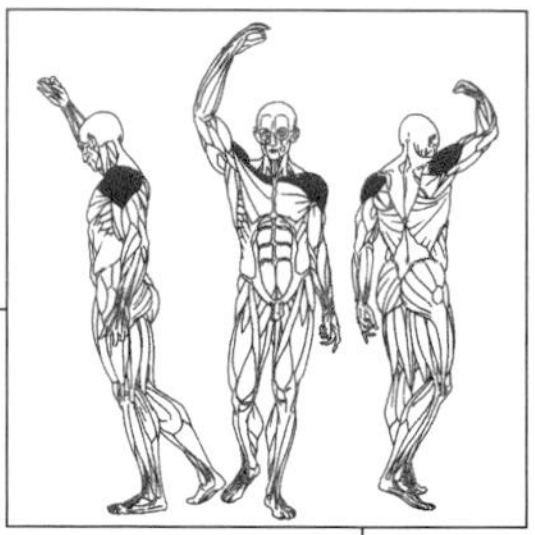

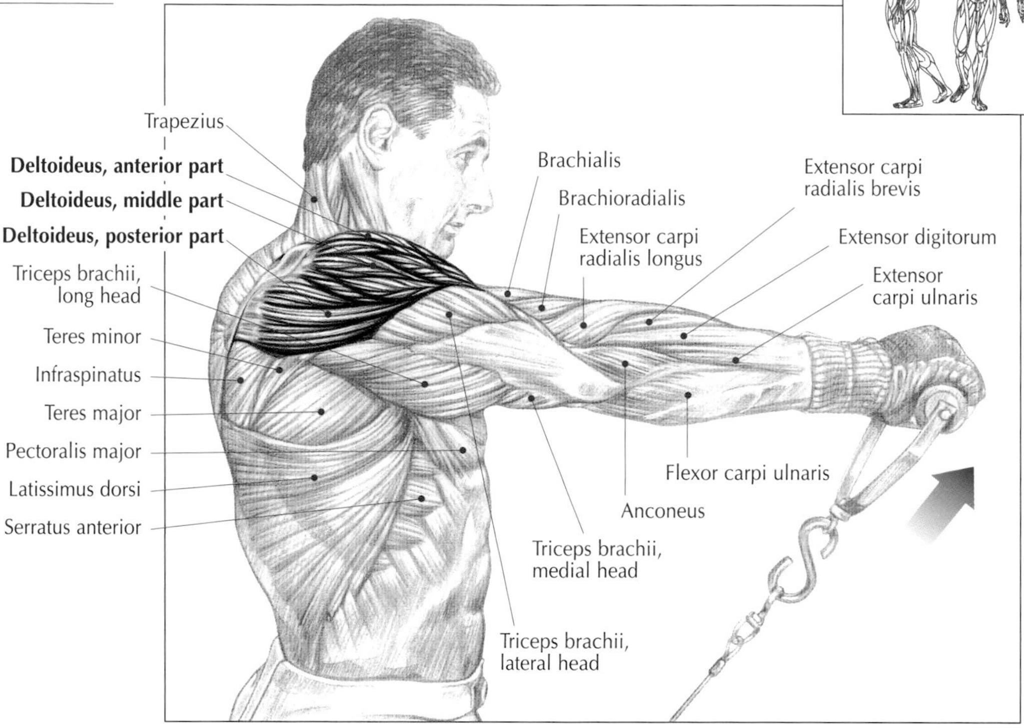

Trapezius

Deltoideus, anterior part

Deltoideus, middle part

Deltoideus, posterior part

Triceps brachii, long head

Teres minor

Infraspinatus

Teres major

Pectoralis major

Latissimus dorsi

Serratus anterior

Brachialis

Brachioradialis

Extensor carpi radialis longus

Extensor carpi radialis brevis

Extensor digitorum

Extensor carpi ulnaris

Flexor carpi ulnaris

Anconeus

Triceps brachii, medial head

Triceps brachii, lateral head

Stand with your feet slightly spread. Hold the handle with an overhand grip, keeping your arms at your sides:
– Inhale and raise your arm forward to shoulder height
– Exhale as you complete the movement

This exercise works the deltoids (particularly the anterior deltoids) as well as the upper pectorals and, to a lesser extent, the short head of the biceps.

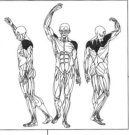

LOW PULLEY BENT-OVER LATERAL RAISES

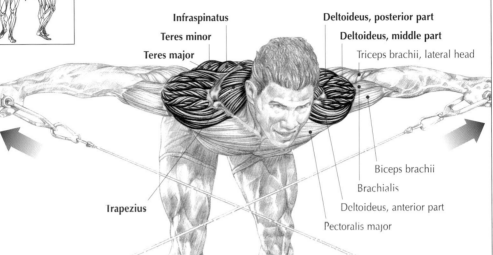

Infraspinatus

Teres minor

Teres major

Deltoideus, posterior part

Deltoideus, middle part

Triceps brachii, lateral head

Biceps brachii

Brachialis

Deltoideus, anterior part

Pectoralis major

Trapezius

Stand with your feet spread and your knees slighlty bent. Bend forward at the waist, keeping your back straight and your arms hanging down. Hold a handle in each hand with the cables crossing each other:
– Inhale and raise your arms to the sides until your hands are slightly above the level of your shoulders
– Exhale as you complete the movement

This exercise works the deltoids, especially the posterior deltoids. At the end of the movement, when you pinch your scapulae together, you emphasize the trapezius (medial and inferior portions) and the rhomboids.

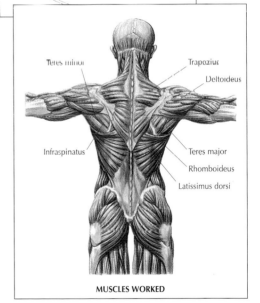

Teres minor

Infraspinatus

Trapezius

Deltoideus

Teres major

Rhomboideus

Latissimus dorsi

MUSCLES WORKED

12 ONE-DUMBBELL FRONT RAISES

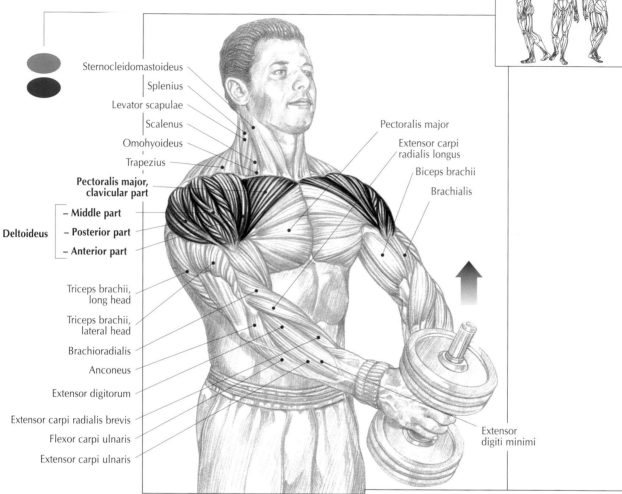

Sternocleidomastoideus

Splenius

Levator scapulae

Scalenus

Omohyoideus

Trapezius

Pectoralis major, clavicular part

Deltoideus
- **Middle part**
- **Posterior part**
- **Anterior part**

Triceps brachii, long head

Triceps brachii, lateral head

Brachioradialis

Anconeus

Extensor digitorum

Extensor carpi radialis brevis

Flexor carpi ulnaris

Extensor carpi ulnaris

Pectoralis major

Extensor carpi radialis longus

Biceps brachii

Brachialis

Extensor digiti minimi

Stand with your feet slightly spread. Keep your back straight and your abdominals contracted. Hold the dumbbell, palms facing in, with your hands overlapping each other. Rest the dumbbell on your thighs with your arms straight:
– Inhale and raise the dumbbell forward until it reaches shoulder level
– Slowly lower the dumbbell, making sure to avoid any jerky movements
– Exhale as you complete the movement

This exercise works the anterior deltoids as well as the upper pectorals and the short head of the biceps.
All the muscles that stabilize the scapulae use isometric action, allowing the humerus to pivot on a stable support.

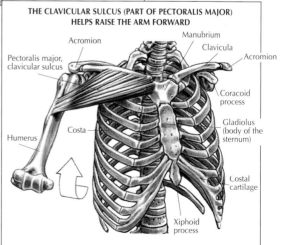

THE CLAVICULAR SULCUS (PART OF PECTORALIS MAJOR) HELPS RAISE THE ARM FORWARD

Acromion

Manubrium

Clavicula

Acromion

Pectoralis major, clavicular sulcus

Coracoid process

Humerus

Costa

Gladiolus (body of the sternum)

Costal cartilage

Xiphoid process

BARBELL FRONT RAISES 13

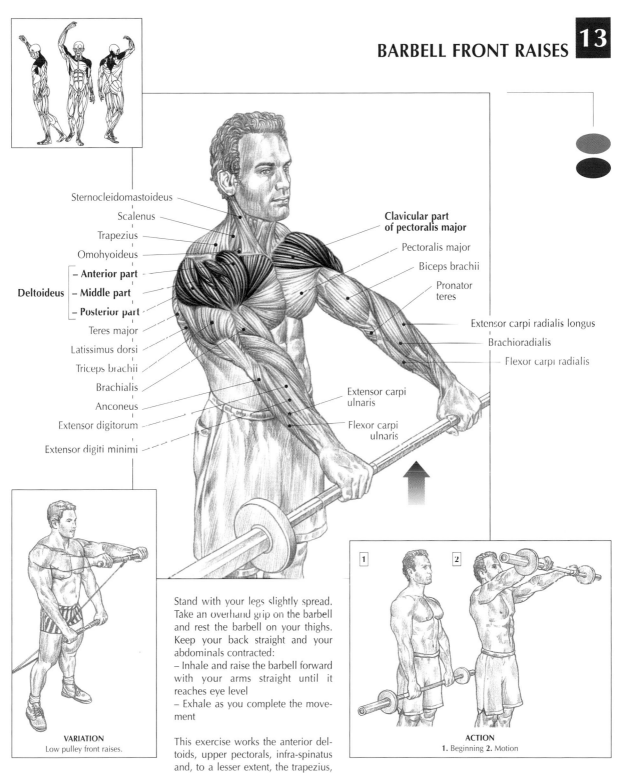

Sternocleidomastoideus

Scalenus

Trapezius

Omohyoideus

Deltoideus – **Anterior part**
– **Middle part**
– **Posterior part**

Teres major

Latissimus dorsi

Triceps brachii

Brachialis

Anconeus

Extensor digitorum

Extensor digiti minimi

**Clavicular part
of pectoralis major**

Pectoralis major

Biceps brachii

Pronator
teres

Extensor carpi radialis longus

Brachioradialis

Flexor carpi radialis

Extensor carpi
ulnaris

Flexor carpi
ulnaris

VARIATION
Low pulley front raises.

Stand with your legs slightly spread.
Take an overhand grip on the barbell
and rest the barbell on your thighs.
Keep your back straight and your
abdominals contracted:
– Inhale and raise the barbell forward
with your arms straight until it
reaches eye level
– Exhale as you complete the movement

This exercise works the anterior deltoids, upper pectorals, infra-spinatus
and, to a lesser extent, the trapezius,

ACTION
1. Beginning **2.** Motion

serratus anterior, and short head of the biceps. If you raise the barbell higher, you also stress the posterior deltoids. Doing so intensifies the
work of the other muscles. The same exercise can be performed with a low pulley machine while facing away from the machine with the
cable running between your legs.
Note: every front raise arm exercise places secondary emphasis on the biceps.

14 UPRIGHT ROWS

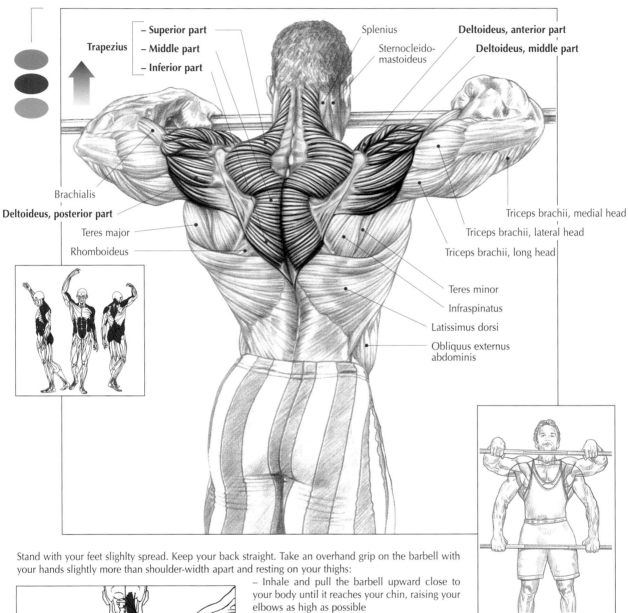

Trapezius
– **Superior part**
– **Middle part**
– **Inferior part**

Splenius

Sternocleido-mastoideus

Deltoideus, anterior part

Deltoideus, middle part

Brachialis

Deltoideus, posterior part

Teres major

Rhomboideus

Triceps brachii, medial head

Triceps brachii, lateral head

Triceps brachii, long head

Teres minor

Infraspinatus

Latissimus dorsi

Obliquus externus abdominis

ACTION

Stand with your feet slightly spread. Keep your back straight. Take an overhand grip on the barbell with your hands slightly more than shoulder-width apart and resting on your thighs:

– Inhale and pull the barbell upward close to your body until it reaches your chin, raising your elbows as high as possible
– Slowly return to the arms-extended position, avoiding any jerky movements
– Exhale as you complete the movement

This exercise directly works the deltoids, trapezius, and biceps, and places secondary emphasis on the forearm, sacrospinalis, and abdominal muscles.

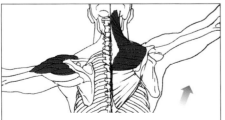

Once the deltoid moves the arm upward in a horizontal position, the trapezius takes over to move the scapula, allowing you to raise your arm higher.

NAUTILUS LATERAL RAISES 15

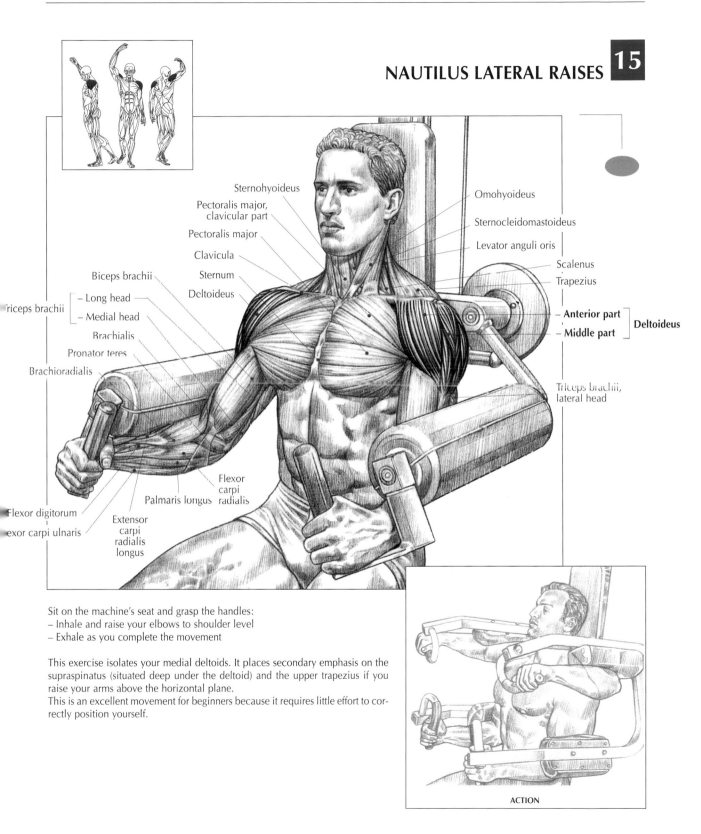

Sternohyoideus
Pectoralis major, clavicular part
Pectoralis major
Clavicula
Sternum
Deltoideus
Biceps brachii
Triceps brachii
– Long head
– Medial head
Brachialis
Pronator teres
Brachioradialis
Omohyoideus
Sternocleidomastoideus
Levator anguli oris
Scalenus
Trapezius
– **Anterior part**
– **Middle part** **Deltoideus**
Triceps brachii, lateral head
Flexor carpi radialis
Palmaris longus
Flexor digitorum
Flexor carpi ulnaris
Extensor carpi radialis longus

Sit on the machine's seat and grasp the handles:
– Inhale and raise your elbows to shoulder level
– Exhale as you complete the movement

This exercise isolates your medial deltoids. It places secondary emphasis on the supraspinatus (situated deep under the deltoid) and the upper trapezius if you raise your arms above the horizontal plane.
This is an excellent movement for beginners because it requires little effort to correctly position yourself.

ACTION

39

16 PEC DECK REAR DELT LATERALS

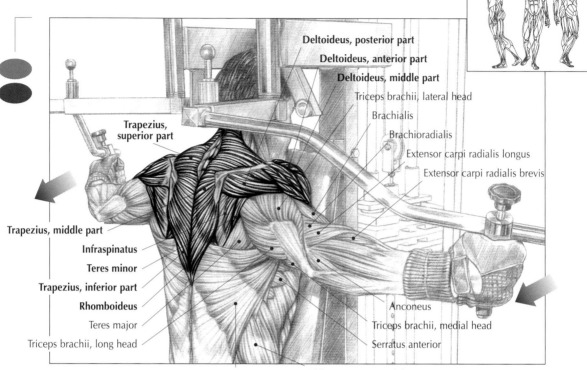

Deltoideus, posterior part
Deltoideus, anterior part
Deltoideus, middle part
Triceps brachii, lateral head
Brachialis
Brachioradialis
Extensor carpi radialis longus
Extensor carpi radialis brevis

Trapezius, superior part

Trapezius, middle part
Infraspinatus
Teres minor
Trapezius, inferior part
Rhomboideus
Teres major
Triceps brachii, long head

Anconeus
Triceps brachii, medial head
Serratus anterior

Latissimus dorsi
Obliquus externus abdominis

ACTION

Sit in a pec deck machine facing toward its back support with your arms stretched out grasping the handles:
– Inhale and force your elbows to the rear, pressing your scapulae together at the end of the movement
– Exhale as you complete the movement

This exercise works
– the deltoids, particularly the posterior part ;
– the infraspinatus; and
– the teres minor.
At the end of the movement, when you pinch your scapulae together, it also works
– the trapezius and
– the rhomboids.

3 CHEST

1. Bench Press
2. Close-Grip Bench Press
3. Incline Press
4. Decline Press
5. Push-Ups
6. Parallel Bar Dips
7. Dumbbell Press
8. Dumbbell Flys
9. Incline Dumbbell Press
10. Incline Dumbbell Flys
11. Pec Deck Flys
12. Cable Crossover Flys
13. Dumbbell Pullovers
14. Barbell Pullovers

1 BENCH PRESS

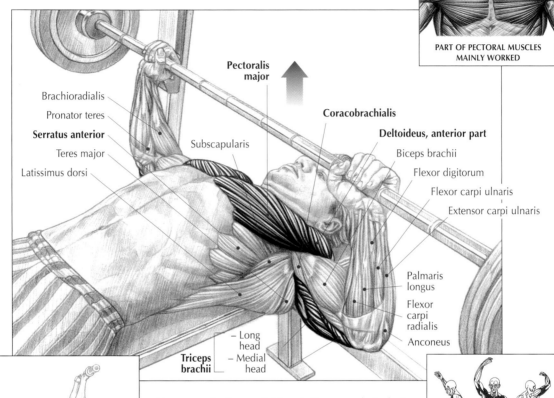

PART OF PECTORAL MUSCLES
MAINLY WORKED

Brachioradialis
Pronator teres
Serratus anterior
Teres major
Latissimus dorsi

Pectoralis major

Subscapularis

Coracobrachialis

Deltoideus, anterior part

Biceps brachii
Flexor digitorum
Flexor carpi ulnaris
Extensor carpi ulnaris

Palmaris longus
Flexor carpi radialis
Anconeus

– Long head
– Medial head

Triceps brachii

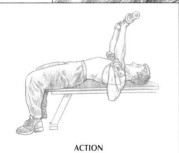

ACTION

Lie on your back on a flat bench. Keep your buttocks in contact with the bench and your feet flat on the floor:
– Take an overhand grip on the barbell with your hands more than shoulder-width apart
– Inhale and slowly lower the barbell until it reaches your chest
– Press the weight back up, exhaling as you complete the movement

This exercise focuses on the pectorals and places secondary emphasis on the triceps, anterior deltoids, serratus, and coracobrachialis.

Variations :
1. Arch your back to work the more powerful lower pectorals and lift heavier loads. However, perform this variation carefully to reduce the likelihood of injury to your back.
2. Press the barbell with your elbows at your sides to focus more on the anterior deltoids.
3. Vary the width of your grip:
– A narrow grip shifts the focus to the inner pectorals
– A very wide grip shifts the focus to the outer pectorals
4. Lower the bar
– to the lower chest (near the edge of the rib cage) to work the lower pectorals;
– to the middle of the chest to work the medial pectorals; and
– to the upper chest/lower neck area to work the upper pectorals.
5. Raise your feet from the floor by curling your legs over your abdominals if you have back problems or if you want to place more emphasis on the pectorals.
6. Use a Smith-machine.

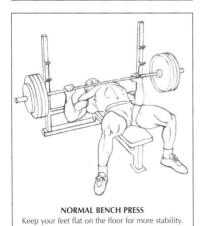

NORMAL BENCH PRESS
Keep your feet flat on the floor for more stability.

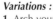

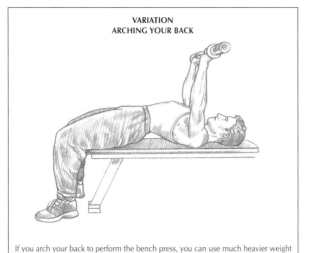

**VARIATION
ARCHING YOUR BACK**

If you arch your back to perform the bench press, you can use much heavier weight because you will place much more stress on the lower pectorals.
At competition level, you must not move your feet and head. In addition, your buttocks should always remain in contact with the bench.

People who have back problems must avoid this variation.

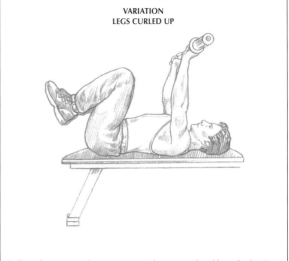

**VARIATION
LEGS CURLED UP**

Curl your legs over your lower torso to avoid extreme arch and lower back pain. This variation can also be used to decrease the emphasis on the lower pectorals, shifting it to the medial and upper pectorals.

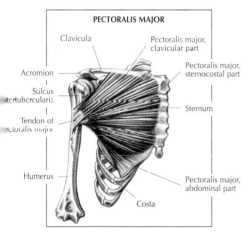

PECTORALIS MAJOR

Clavicula — Pectoralis major, clavicular part — Acromion — Sulcus intertubercularis — Tendon of pectoralis major — Humerus — Pectoralis major, sternocostal part — Sternum — Pectoralis major, abdominal part — Costa

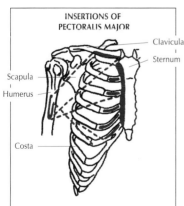

INSERTIONS OF PECTORALIS MAJOR

Clavicula — Sternum — Scapula — Humerus — Costa

Variation with a machine :
Stand or sit, depending on the machine, and grasp the bar or the handles:
– Inhale and press
– Exhale at the end of the movement

This safe exercise is excellent for beginners. It focuses on the pectorals and keeps your body set in the prescribed movement pattern. Beginners can gain strength this way before trying the free weight bench press.
Depending on the type of machine, this exercise allows advanced bodybuilders to isolate the work on the upper, medial, or lower pectorals, helping them develop muscle balance.

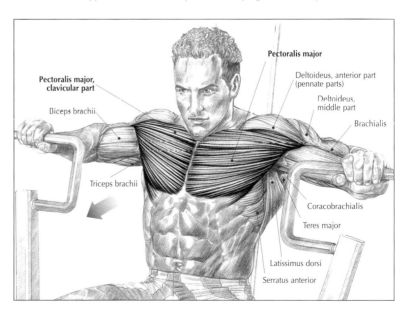

2 CLOSE-GRIP BENCH PRESS

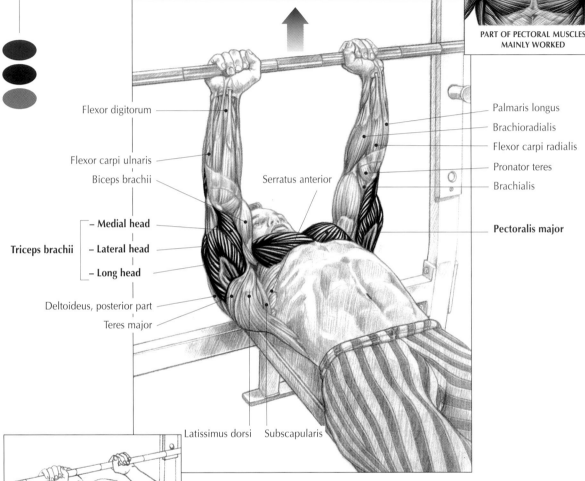

PART OF PECTORAL MUSCLES
MAINLY WORKED

Flexor digitorum

Flexor carpi ulnaris

Biceps brachii

Serratus anterior

Palmaris longus

Brachioradialis

Flexor carpi radialis

Pronator teres

Brachialis

Triceps brachii

– Medial head

– Lateral head

– Long head

Pectoralis major

Deltoideus, posterior part

Teres major

Latissimus dorsi   Subscapularis

**ELBOWS TO THE SIDES TO PLACE MORE
EMPHASIS ON THE TRICEPS**

Lie on your back on a flat bench, keeping your buttocks in contact with the bench and your feet flat on the floor. Take an overhand grip on the barbell with your hands from 4 to 15 inches apart, depending on your wrist flexibility:
– Inhale and slowly lower the barbell until it reaches your chest, allowing your elbows to extend away from your torso
– Press the barbell upward, exhaling as you complete the movement

This exercise is excellent for developing the pectorals and the triceps (for this reason, you can include this exercise in an arm-specific program).
Keep your elbows in if you want to shift the emphasis to the anterior deltoids. You can perform this movement with a Smith-machine.

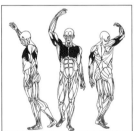

INCLINE PRESS 3

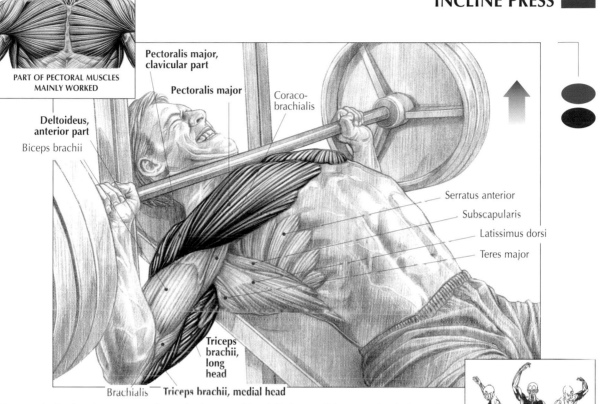

PART OF PECTORAL MUSCLES
MAINLY WORKED

Pectoralis major,
clavicular part

Pectoralis major

Coraco-
brachialis

Deltoideus,
anterior part

Biceps brachii

Serratus anterior

Subscapularis

Latissimus dorsi

Teres major

Triceps
brachii,
long
head

Brachialis   Triceps brachii, medial head

Lie on an incline bench set at an angle ranging between 45 and 60 degrees. Take an overhand grip on the barbell with your hands more than shoulder-width apart:
– Inhale and lower the barbell until it reaches your jugular notch (upper chest at the base of your neck)
– Press the bar back up to straight arms length, exhaling as you complete the movement

This exercise works the upper pectorals, anterior deltoids, triceps, and serratus anterior.
You can use a weight rack to perform this movement.

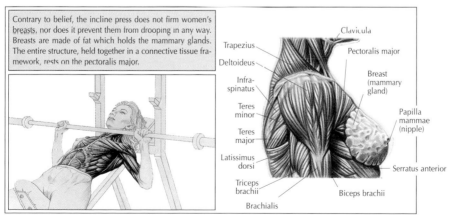

Contrary to belief, the incline press does not firm women's breasts, nor does it prevent them from drooping in any way. Breasts are made of fat which holds the mammary glands. The entire structure, held together in a connective tissue framework, rests on the pectoralis major.

Clavicula

Trapezius

Pectoralis major

Deltoideus

Breast
(mammary
gland)

Infra-
spinatus

Teres
minor

Papilla
mammae
(nipple)

Teres
major

Latissimus
dorsi

Serratus anterior

Triceps
brachii

Biceps brachii

Brachialis

4 DECLINE PRESS

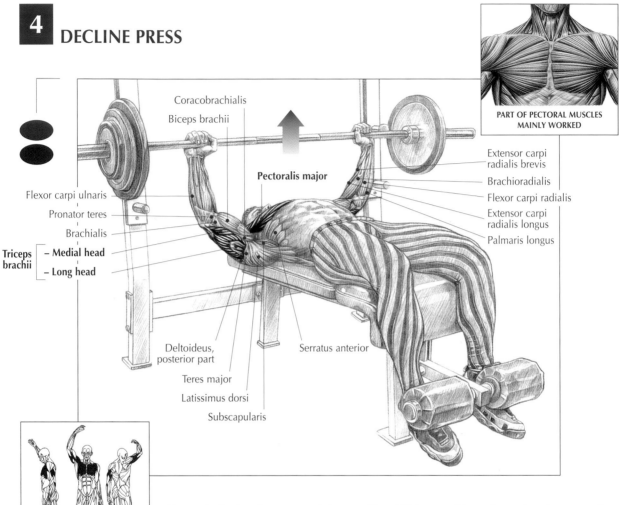

PART OF PECTORAL MUSCLES
MAINLY WORKED

Coracobrachialis

Biceps brachii

Pectoralis major

Flexor carpi ulnaris

Pronator teres

Brachialis

Triceps brachii
– Medial head
– Long head

Extensor carpi radialis brevis

Brachioradialis

Flexor carpi radialis

Extensor carpi radialis longus

Palmaris longus

Deltoideus, posterior part

Serratus anterior

Teres major

Latissimus dorsi

Subscapularis

Lie on a decline bench set at an angle between 20 and 40 degrees with your feet anchored to prevent them from slipping. Take an overhand grip on the bar with your hands at least shoulder-width apart:
– Inhale and slowly lower the bar until it reaches the lower edge of your pectorals
– Press the bar back up, exhaling as you complete the movement

This exercise works the pectoralis major (particularly the lower part), triceps, and anterior deltoids. It places secondary emphasis on the lower fold of the pectorals. In addition, lowering the bar to neck level helps stretch the pectoralis major, increasing its flexibility.
You can also use a Smith-machine.

PUSH-UPS 5

PART OF PECTORAL MUSCLES MAINLY WORKED

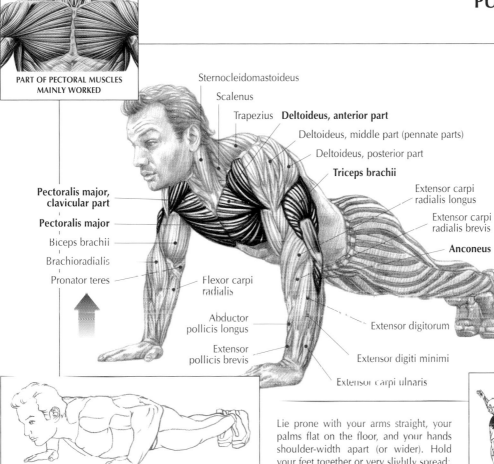

Sternocleidomastoideus

Scalenus

Trapezius   **Deltoideus, anterior part**

Deltoideus, middle part (pennate parts)

Deltoideus, posterior part

Triceps brachii

Extensor carpi radialis longus

Extensor carpi radialis brevis

Anconeus

Pectoralis major, clavicular part

Pectoralis major

Biceps brachii

Brachioradialis

Pronator teres

Flexor carpi radialis

Abductor pollicis longus

Extensor pollicis brevis

Extensor digitorum

Extensor digiti minimi

Extensor carpi ulnaris

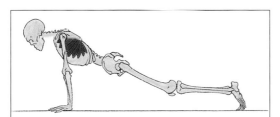

STARTING POSITION

When you do push-ups, the contraction of the serratus anterior holds the scapulae on the rib cage, combining arm and torso action.

Lie prone with your arms straight, your palms flat on the floor, and your hands shoulder-width apart (or wider). Hold your feet together or very slightly spread:
– Inhale and bend your elbows to bring your torso near the floor, avoiding extreme hyperextension of your spine
  Push yourself back to an arms-extended position, exhaling as you complete the movement

This exercise is excellent for developing the pectoralis major and the triceps. You can do it anywhere.
Vary the torso angle to isolate the work:
– Elevate the feet to focus on the upper pectorals
– Elevate the torso to focus on the lower pectorals

6 PARALLEL BAR DIPS

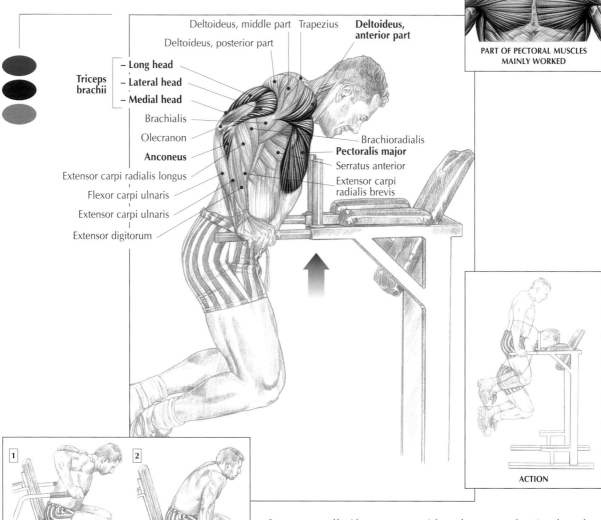

Deltoideus, middle part

Trapezius

Deltoideus, anterior part

Deltoideus, posterior part

PART OF PECTORAL MUSCLES MAINLY WORKED

Triceps brachii
- **– Long head**
- **– Lateral head**
- **– Medial head**

Brachialis

Olecranon

Anconeus

Extensor carpi radialis longus

Flexor carpi ulnaris

Extensor carpi ulnaris

Extensor digitorum

Brachioradialis

Pectoralis major

Serratus anterior

Extensor carpi radialis brevis

ACTION

DIPS WITH MACHINE
1. Beginning of movement 2. End of movement

Support yourself with your arms straight and your torso hanging down from your shoulders:
– Inhale and bend your elbows to allow your body to sink as far down between the bars as possible
– Reverse the motion and return to the starting point, exhaling as you complete the movement

The more you bend forward, the more you work the pectorals. Conversely, the more you straighten your torso, the more you involve the triceps.

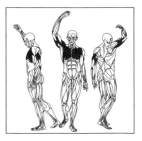

This exercise is excellent for stretching the pectoralis major and increasing the flexibility of the pectoral girdle. However, it is not recommended to beginners because it requires sufficient strength. To that purpose, use the machine to master the technique.

Sets of 10 to 20 reps give the best results. To gain more power and size, experienced athletes can hang a dumbbell between their legs or place barbell plates around their waist.

Note: always perform the dips carefully to avoid traumatizing the shoulder joint.

DUMBBELL PRESS 7

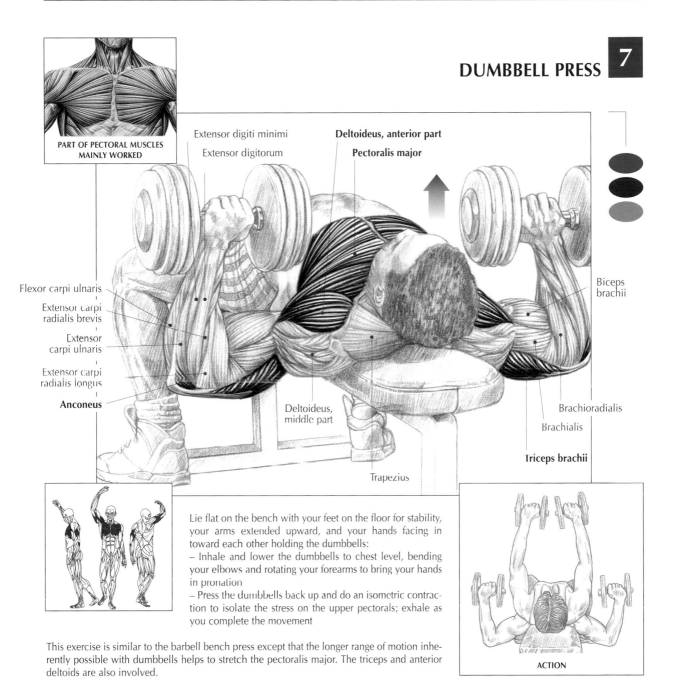

PART OF PECTORAL MUSCLES
MAINLY WORKED

Extensor digiti minimi

Extensor digitorum

Deltoideus, anterior part

Pectoralis major

Flexor carpi ulnaris

Extensor carpi
radialis brevis

Extensor
carpi ulnaris

Extensor carpi
radialis longus

Anconeus

Deltoideus,
middle part

Trapezius

Biceps
brachii

Brachioradialis

Brachialis

Triceps brachii

Lie flat on the bench with your feet on the floor for stability, your arms extended upward, and your hands facing in toward each other holding the dumbbells:
– Inhale and lower the dumbbells to chest level, bending your elbows and rotating your forearms to bring your hands in pronation
– Press the dumbbells back up and do an isometric contraction to isolate the stress on the upper pectorals; exhale as you complete the movement

ACTION

This exercise is similar to the barbell bench press except that the longer range of motion inherently possible with dumbbells helps to stretch the pectoralis major. The triceps and anterior deltoids are also involved.

8 DUMBBELL FLYS

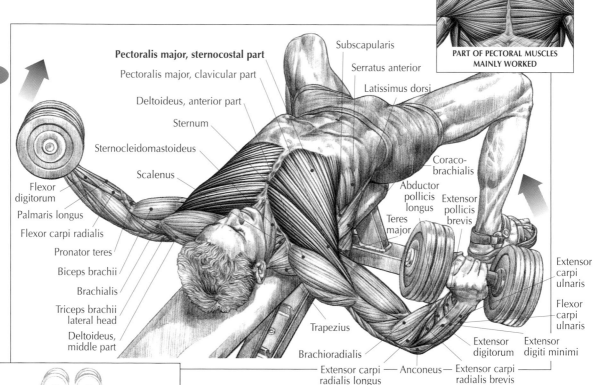

Pectoralis major, sternocostal part

Pectoralis major, clavicular part

Deltoideus, anterior part

Sternum

Sternocleidomastoideus

Scalenus

Flexor digitorum

Palmaris longus

Flexor carpi radialis

Pronator teres

Biceps brachii

Brachialis

Triceps brachii lateral head

Deltoideus, middle part

Subscapularis

Serratus anterior

Latissimus dorsi

Coraco-brachialis

Abductor pollicis longus

Teres major

Extensor pollicis brevis

Extensor carpi ulnaris

Flexor carpi ulnaris

Extensor digiti minimi

Extensor digitorum

Extensor carpi radialis brevis

Anconeus

Trapezius

Brachioradialis

Extensor carpi radialis longus

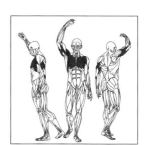

PART OF PECTORAL MUSCLES MAINLY WORKED

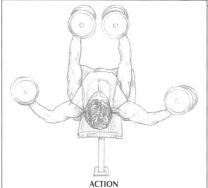

ACTION

Lie flat on a narrow bench to allow free movement of your shoulders. Hold the dumbbells with your arms extended and your elbows slightly bent to lessen the stress on the joint:
– Inhale, then lower the dumbbells until your elbows are at shoulder height
– Raise the dumbbells back up while exhaling
– Perform a short isometric contraction at the end of the movement to place more focus on the upper pectorals (sternal part)

This exercise should never be performed with heavy weight. It isolates the pectoralis major and is an excellent movement for improving flexibility.

INCLINE DUMBBELL PRESS **9**

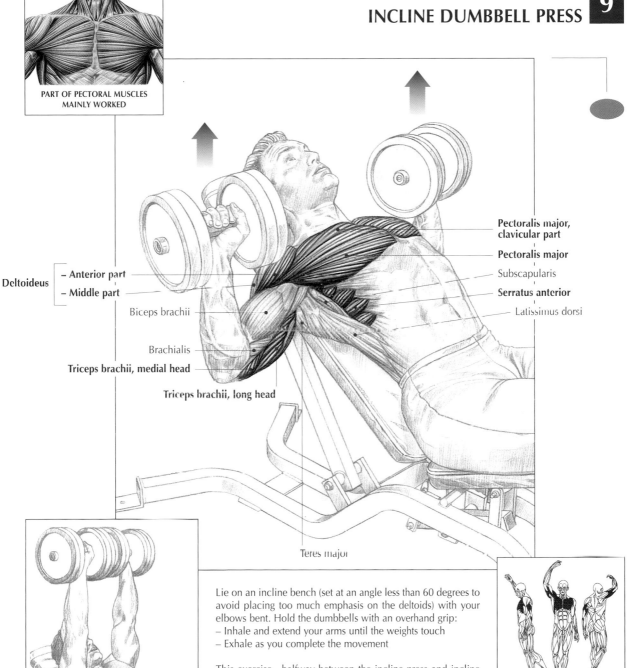

PART OF PECTORAL MUSCLES
MAINLY WORKED

Deltoideus

– Anterior part
– Middle part

Biceps brachii

Brachialis

Triceps brachii, medial head

Triceps brachii, long head

Pectoralis major,
clavicular part

Pectoralis major

Subscapularis

Serratus anterior

Latissimus dorsi

Teres major

END OF MOVEMENT

Lie on an incline bench (set at an angle less than 60 degrees to avoid placing too much emphasis on the deltoids) with your elbows bent. Hold the dumbbells with an overhand grip:
– Inhale and extend your arms until the weights touch
– Exhale as you complete the movement

This exercise—halfway between the incline press and incline dumbbell flys—works the pectorals (particularly the upper part) while stretching them. It also works the anterior deltoids, serratus anterior, and pectoralis minor (both stabilize the scapulae, allowing the arm to work with the torso), and the triceps.

Variation: to isolate the effort on the upper pectorals, start the movement with an overhand grip and rotate your wrists so the dumbbells face each other.

10 INCLINE DUMBBELL FLYS

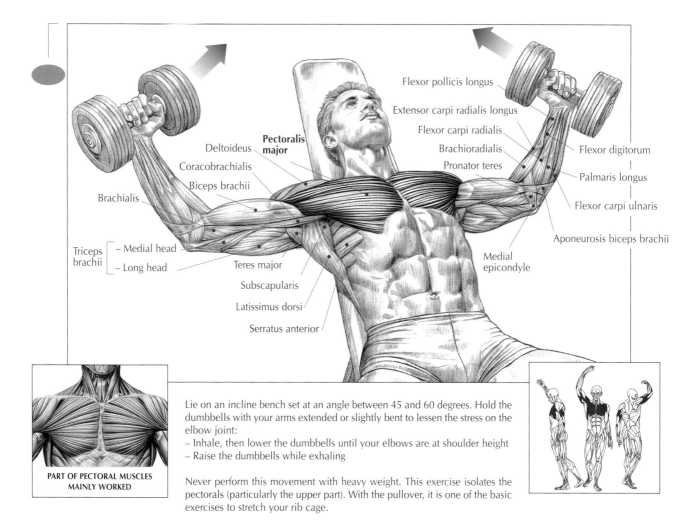

Flexor pollicis longus
Extensor carpi radialis longus
Flexor carpi radialis
Brachioradialis
Pronator teres
Flexor digitorum
Palmaris longus
Flexor carpi ulnaris
Aponeurosis biceps brachii
Medial epicondyle

Pectoralis major
Deltoideus
Coracobrachialis
Biceps brachii
Brachialis
Triceps brachii — Medial head
— Long head
Teres major
Subscapularis
Latissimus dorsi
Serratus anterior

PART OF PECTORAL MUSCLES MAINLY WORKED

Lie on an incline bench set at an angle between 45 and 60 degrees. Hold the dumbbells with your arms extended or slightly bent to lessen the stress on the elbow joint:
– Inhale, then lower the dumbbells until your elbows are at shoulder height
– Raise the dumbbells while exhaling

Never perform this movement with heavy weight. This exercise isolates the pectorals (particularly the upper part). With the pullover, it is one of the basic exercises to stretch your rib cage.

PEC DECK FLYS 11

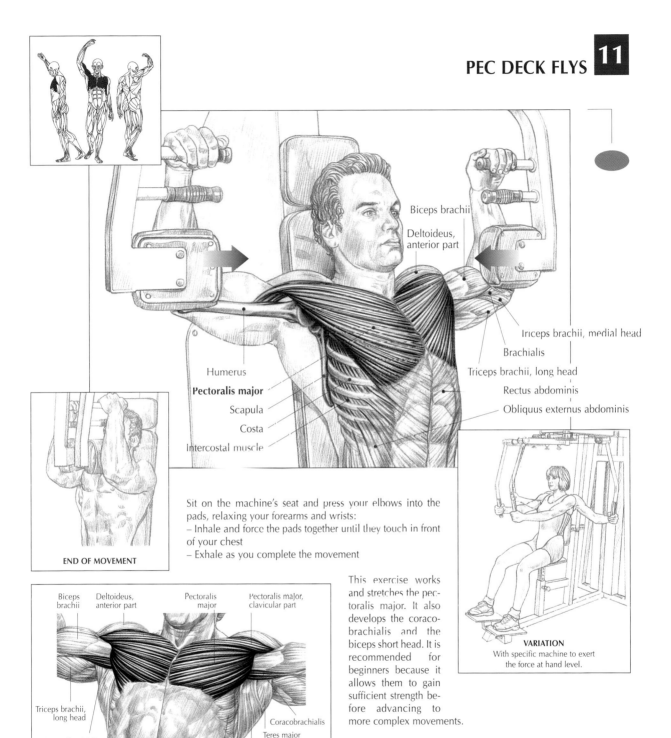

Biceps brachii

Deltoideus, anterior part

Triceps brachii, medial head

Brachialis

Triceps brachii, long head

Rectus abdominis

Obliquus externus abdominis

Humerus

Pectoralis major

Scapula

Costa

Intercostal muscle

END OF MOVEMENT

Biceps brachii

Deltoideus, anterior part

Pectoralis major

Pectoralis major, clavicular part

Triceps brachii, long head

Coracobrachialis

Coracobrachialis

Teres major

Latissimus dorsi

Sternum   Serratus anterior   Subscapularis

Sit on the machine's seat and press your elbows into the pads, relaxing your forearms and wrists:
– Inhale and force the pads together until they touch in front of your chest
– Exhale as you complete the movement

This exercise works and stretches the pectoralis major. It also develops the coracobrachialis and the biceps short head. It is recommended for beginners because it allows them to gain sufficient strength before advancing to more complex movements.

VARIATION
With specific machine to exert the force at hand level.

12 CABLE CROSSOVER FLYS

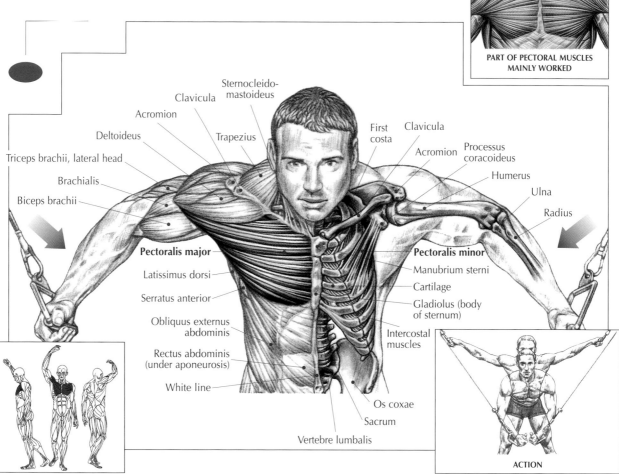

PART OF PECTORAL MUSCLES
MAINLY WORKED

Sternocleido-
mastoideus

Clavicula

Acromion

Deltoideus

Trapezius

First
costa

Clavicula

Acromion

Processus
coracoideus

Humerus

Triceps brachii, lateral head

Brachialis

Biceps brachii

Ulna

Radius

Pectoralis major

Latissimus dorsi

Serratus anterior

Obliquus externus
abdominis

Rectus abdominis
(under aponeurosis)

White line

Pectoralis minor

Manubrium sterni

Cartilage

Gladiolus (body
of sternum)

Intercostal
muscles

Os coxae

Sacrum

Vertebre lumbalis

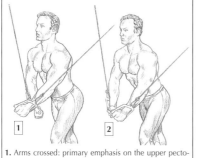

ACTION

Stand with your feet slightly spread, your body slightly forward, and your elbows slightly bent. Hold the handles with your arms spread:
– Inhale and press the cable handles forward until your hands touch
– Exhale as you complete the contraction

This is an excellent exercise for the pectorals. You can vary the tilt of your torso and the angle of your arms to stress the entire pectoralis major.

Note: cable crossover flys also involve the pectoralis minor under the pectoralis major. Besides stabilizing the scapulae, the pectoralis minor functions to protract the shoulder.

1. Arms crossed: primary emphasis on the upper pectorals at the end of movement **2.** Normal action

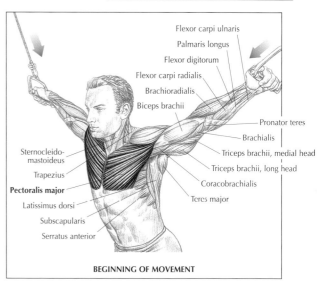

Flexor carpi ulnaris

Palmaris longus

Flexor digitorum

Flexor carpi radialis

Brachioradialis

Biceps brachii

Pronator teres

Brachialis

Triceps brachii, medial head

Triceps brachii, long head

Coracobrachialis

Teres major

Sternocleido-
mastoideus

Trapezius

Pectoralis major

Latissimus dorsi

Subscapularis

Serratus anterior

BEGINNING OF MOVEMENT

DUMBBELL PULLOVERS 13

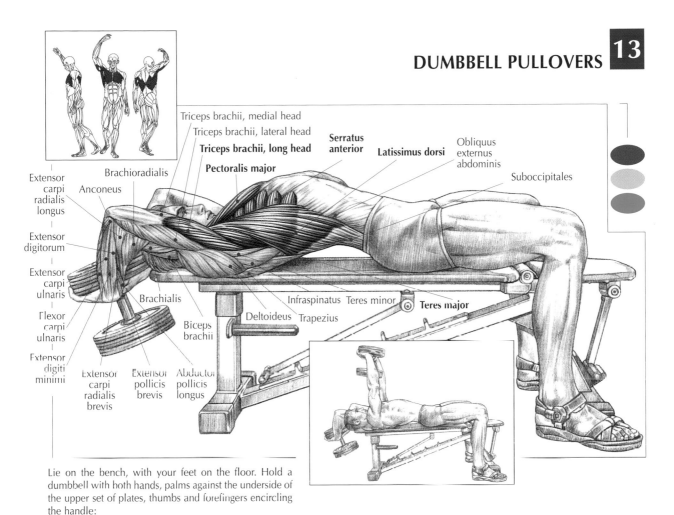

Triceps brachii, medial head
Triceps brachii, lateral head
Triceps brachii, long head
Pectoralis major
Serratus anterior
Latissimus dorsi
Obliquus externus abdominis
Suboccipitales
Brachioradialis
Extensor carpi radialis longus
Anconeus
Extensor digitorum
Extensor carpi ulnaris
Flexor carpi ulnaris
Extensor digiti minimi
Brachialis
Biceps brachii
Extensor carpi radialis brevis
Extensor pollicis brevis
Abductor pollicis longus
Deltoideus
Trapezius
Infraspinatus
Teres minor
Teres major

Lie on the bench, with your feet on the floor. Hold a dumbbell with both hands, palms against the underside of the upper set of plates, thumbs and forefingers encircling the handle:
– Inhale as you lower the weight behind your head, slightly bending your elbows
– Return to the starting position, exhaling

This exercise develops the entire pectoral muscle and works the triceps long head, teres major, lats, serratus anterior, rhomboids, and pectoralis minor. You can do this movement to stretch your rib cage. To do so, use a light dumbbell and make sure you bend your elbows slightly. If possible, use a convex bench or lie across a flat bench with your pelvis lower than your pectoral girdle. It is best to inhale as much as possible when you start the movement and to exhale only as you raise the dumbbell.

SCAPULA STABILIZERS

Trapezius
Cranium
Vertebra
Levator scapulae
Levator scapulae
Clavicula
Spina scapulae
Acromion
Rhomboideus minor
Pectoralis minor
Rhomboideus major
Sternum
Serratus anterior
Serratus anterior
Costa
Costal cartilage

POSTERIOR   **ANTERIOR**

VARIATION

Lying across a flat bench helps to stretch your rib cage.

MACHINE PULLOVERS

14 BARBELL PULLOVERS

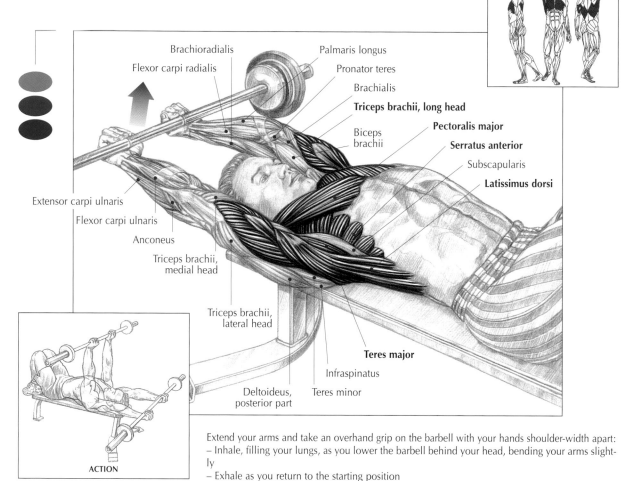

Brachioradialis

Flexor carpi radialis

Palmaris longus

Pronator teres

Brachialis

Triceps brachii, long head

Biceps brachii

Pectoralis major

Serratus anterior

Subscapularis

Latissimus dorsi

Extensor carpi ulnaris

Flexor carpi ulnaris

Anconeus

Triceps brachii, medial head

Triceps brachii, lateral head

Teres major

Infraspinatus

Teres minor

Deltoideus, posterior part

ACTION

Extend your arms and take an overhand grip on the barbell with your hands shoulder-width apart:
– Inhale, filling your lungs, as you lower the barbell behind your head, bending your arms slightly
– Exhale as you return to the starting position

This exercise develops the pectoralis major, triceps long head, teres major, lats, serratus anterior, rhomboids, and pectoralis minor. It is an excellent movement for stretching the rib cage. To do so, use a light barbell and don't forget to position yourself and breathe correctly.

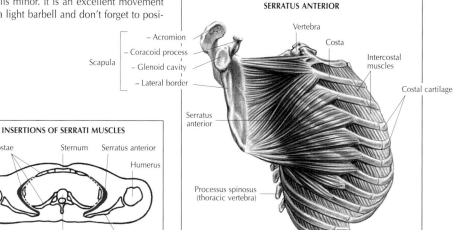

SERRATUS ANTERIOR

Vertebra

Costa

Intercostal muscles

Scapula

– Acromion
– Coracoid process
– Glenoid cavity
– Lateral border

Costal cartilage

Serratus anterior

Processus spinosus (thoracic vertebra)

INSERTIONS OF SERRATI MUSCLES

Costae

Sternum

Serratus anterior

Humerus

Vertebra

Scapula

1. Chin-Ups
2. Reverse Chin-Ups
3. Lat Pulldowns
4. Back Lat Pulldowns
5. Close-Grip Lat Pulldowns
6. Straight-Arm Lat Pulldowns
7. Seated Rows
8. One-Arm Dumbbell Rows
9. Bent Rows
10. T-Bar Rows
11. Stiff-Legged Deadlifts
12. Deadlifts
13. Sumo Deadlifts
14. Back Extension
15. Upright Rows
16. Barbell Shrugs
17. Dumbbell Shrugs
18. Machine Shrugs

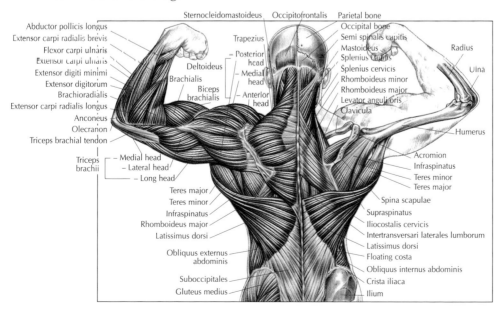

1 CHIN-UPS

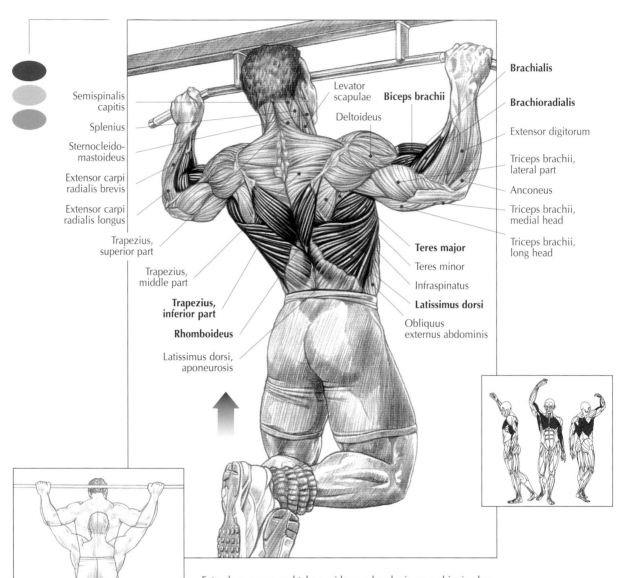

Semispinalis capitis
Splenius
Sternocleido-mastoideus
Extensor carpi radialis brevis
Extensor carpi radialis longus
Trapezius, superior part
Trapezius, middle part
Trapezius, inferior part
Rhomboideus
Latissimus dorsi, aponeurosis

Levator scapulae
Biceps brachii
Deltoideus

Brachialis
Brachioradialis
Extensor digitorum
Triceps brachii, lateral part
Anconeus
Triceps brachii, medial head
Triceps brachii, long head

Teres major
Teres minor
Infraspinatus
Latissimus dorsi
Obliquus externus abdominis

**VARIATION
CHIN-UPS BEHIND THE NECK**

Extend your arms and take a wide, overhand grip on a chinning bar:
– Inhale and pull yourself upward until your eyes are above the level of the bar
– Exhale as you complete the movement

This full-back exercise requires greater strength. It is an excellent movement for working the biceps, brachialis, brachioradialis, and pectoralis major.

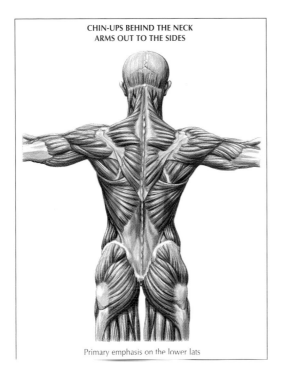

**CHIN-UPS BEHIND THE NECK
ARMS OUT TO THE SIDES**

Primary emphasis on the lower lats

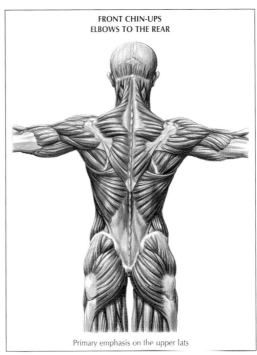

**FRONT CHIN-UPS
ELBOWS TO THE REAR**

Primary emphasis on the upper lats

Variation:
If you stick out your chest, you can pull yourself up so the bar touches your chin. To increase the intensity, you will need added resistance attached to your body. When you pull your elbows to the rear and stick out your chest until your chin reaches the level of the bar, the movement mainly involves the upper and lats, as well as the teres major.

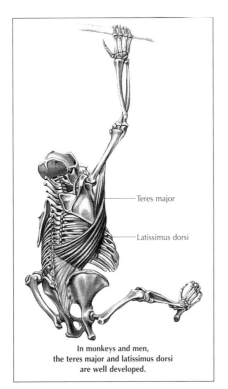

Teres major

Latissimus dorsi

**In monkeys and men,
the teres major and latissimus dorsi
are well developed.**

This exercise adds thickness to the back. When you pinch your scapulae together, the rhomboids and the inferior part of the trapezius are also worked.

EVOLUTIONARY THEORY

Originally, the teres major and latissimus dorsi were involved in making our remote ancestors walk on all fours. They mainly worked on the forelegs as reverse thrusters. With the transition to arboreal life, they became powerful muscles specialized in vertical movement. When our ancestors returned to the ground, they adopted bipedalism but kept their ability to climb trees. For this reason, we still have powerful back muscles that allow us to pull ourselves up and climb trees, walls, ladders, and so forth.

Note: the main difference between our locomotor system and that of the apes lies in the development of our lower limbs, which are specialized for bipedalism. Our chest and upper limbs have quite the same structure and proportions as those of the apes. Contrarily to fallacies, apes don't have long arms: humans have long legs.

2 REVERSE CHIN-UPS

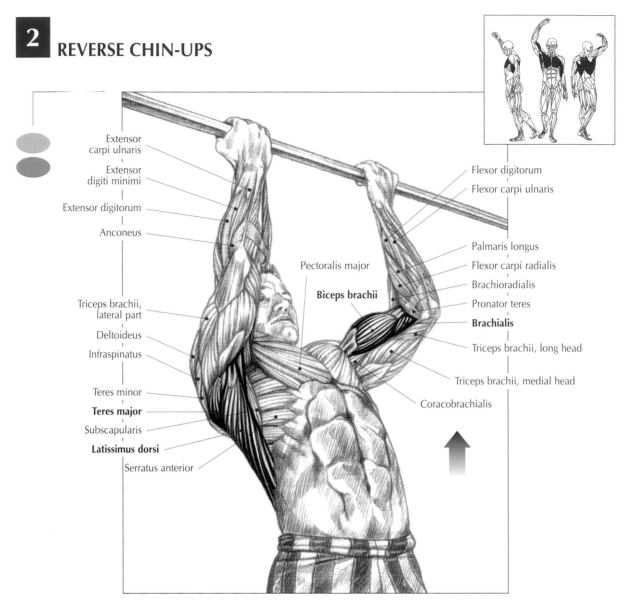

Extensor carpi ulnaris

Extensor digiti minimi

Extensor digitorum

Anconeus

Triceps brachii, lateral part

Deltoideus

Infraspinatus

Teres minor

Teres major

Subscapularis

Latissimus dorsi

Serratus anterior

Pectoralis major

Biceps brachii

Flexor digitorum

Flexor carpi ulnaris

Palmaris longus

Flexor carpi radialis

Brachioradialis

Pronator teres

Brachialis

Triceps brachii, long head

Triceps brachii, medial head

Coracobrachialis

Extend your arms and take an underhand grip on the bar with your hands shoulder-width apart:
– Inhale and stick your chest out to pull yourself upward until your chin is at the level of the bar
– Exhale as you complete the movement

This movement develops the lats and teres major. It places intense focus on the biceps and brachialis. For that reason it can be integrated into a program focused on training the arm region. The trapezius (middle and lower portions), rhomboids, and pectorals are also involved. This exercise requires greater strength. It is easier to perform using a high pulley.

LAT PULLDOWNS 3

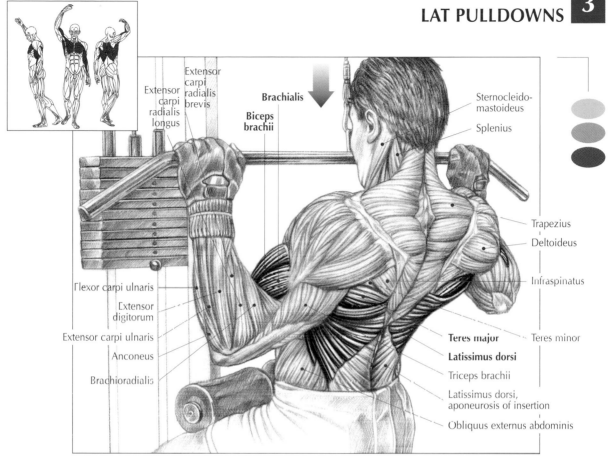

Extensor carpi radialis brevis

Extensor carpi radialis longus

Brachialis

Biceps brachii

Sternocleido-mastoideus

Splenius

Trapezius

Deltoideus

Infraspinatus

Flexor carpi ulnaris

Extensor digitorum

Extensor carpi ulnaris

Anconeus

Brachioradialis

Teres major

Teres minor

Latissimus dorsi

Triceps brachii

Latissimus dorsi, aponeurosis of insertion

Obliquus externus abdominis

Sit facing the machine and wedge your knees under the restraint pad provided. Take a very wide overhand grip on the bar:
– Inhale and pull the bar down to your upper chest, arching your back and bringing your elbows back
– Exhale as you complete the movement
This exercise is excellent for adding thickness to the back. It particularly stresses the center part of the lats. It also places emphasis on the trapezius (middle and lower portions), rhomboids, biceps, brachialis, and, to a lesser extent, on the pectorals.

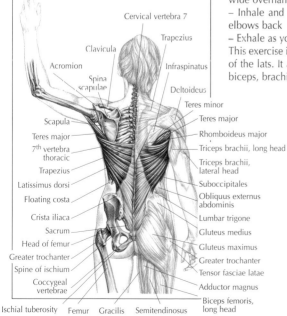

Cervical vertebra 7

Trapezius

Clavicula

Acromion

Spina scapulae

Infraspinatus

Deltoideus

Teres minor

Teres major

Scapula

Rhomboideus major

Teres major

Triceps brachii, long head

7th vertebra thoracic

Triceps brachii, lateral head

Trapezius

Latissimus dorsi

Suboccipitales

Floating costa

Obliquus externus abdominis

Crista iliaca

Lumbar trigone

Sacrum

Gluteus medius

Head of femur

Gluteus maximus

Greater trochanter

Greater trochanter

Spine of ischium

Tensor fasciae latae

Coccygeal vertebrae

Adductor magnus

Biceps femoris, long head

Ischial tuberosity   Femur   Gracilis   Semitendinosus

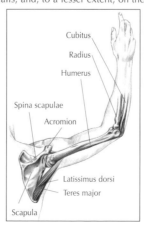

Cubitus

Radius

Humerus

Spina scapulae

Acromion

Latissimus dorsi

Teres major

Scapula

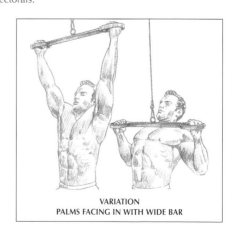

**VARIATION
PALMS FACING IN WITH WIDE BAR**

4 BACK LAT PULLDOWNS

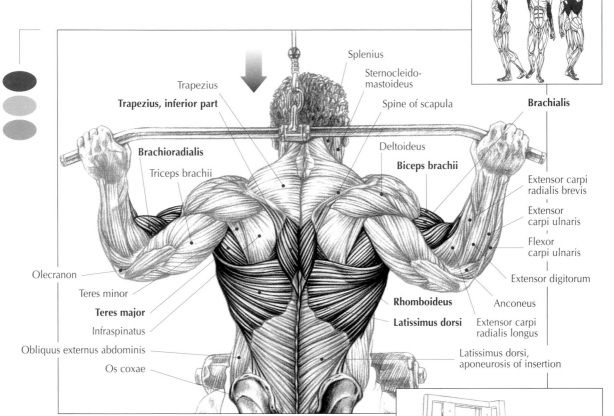

Splenius

Sternocleido-mastoideus

Trapezius

Trapezius, inferior part

Spine of scapula

Deltoideus

Brachialis

Brachioradialis

Triceps brachii

Biceps brachii

Extensor carpi radialis brevis

Extensor carpi ulnaris

Flexor carpi ulnaris

Extensor digitorum

Olecranon

Teres minor

Teres major

Infraspinatus

Obliquus externus abdominis

Os coxae

Rhomboideus

Latissimus dorsi

Anconeus

Extensor carpi radialis longus

Latissimus dorsi, aponeurosis of insertion

Sit facing the machine and secure your thighs under the restraint pad. Take a very wide overhand grip on the bar:
– Inhale and pull the bar down behind your neck, bringing your elbows back as you pull
– Exhale as you complete the movement

This is an excellent exercise for enhancing the back's width. It works the lats, particularly the lower part. It also works the forearm flexor muscles, biceps, brachialis, and brachioradialis in conjunction with the rhomboid and lower trapezius muscles, which work to press the scapulae together.
Lat pulldowns are great for beginners because they allow you to gain strength before trying the chin-ups.

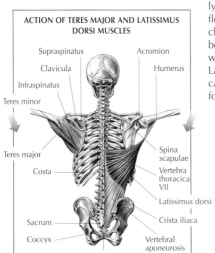

ACTION OF TERES MAJOR AND LATISSIMUS DORSI MUSCLES

Supraspinatus

Clavicula

Infraspinatus

Teres minor

Teres major

Costa

Sacrum

Coccyx

Pubic symphysis

Acromion

Humerus

Spina scapulae

Vertebra thoracica VII

Latissimus dorsi

Crista iliaca

Vertebral aponeurosis

**VARIATION
SPECIFIC MACHINE WITH FIXED AXIS**

CLOSE-GRIP LAT PULLDOWNS 5

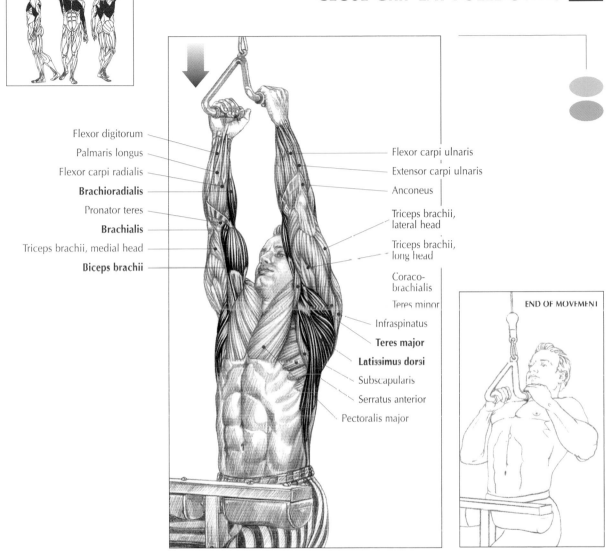

Flexor digitorum
Palmaris longus
Flexor carpi radialis
Brachioradialis
Pronator teres
Brachialis
Triceps brachii, medial head
Biceps brachii

Flexor carpi ulnaris
Extensor carpi ulnaris
Anconeus
Triceps brachii, lateral head
Triceps brachii, long head
Coraco-brachialis
Teres minor
Infraspinatus
Teres major
Latissimus dorsi
Subscapularis
Serratus anterior
Pectoralis major

END OF MOVEMENT

Sit facing the machine and wedge your knees under the restraint pad. Grip the handles with your palms facing toward each other:
– Inhale and pull the handle down to touch the upper part of your chest, arching your back and slightly tilting your upper body backward
– Exhale as you complete the movement

This is an excellent exercise for developing the lats and teres major. When you pinch your scapulae together, you work the rhomboids, trapezius, and posterior deltoids. Every pulldown exercise works the biceps and brachialis and places intense emphasis on the brachioradialis.

6 STRAIGHT-ARM LAT PULLDOWNS

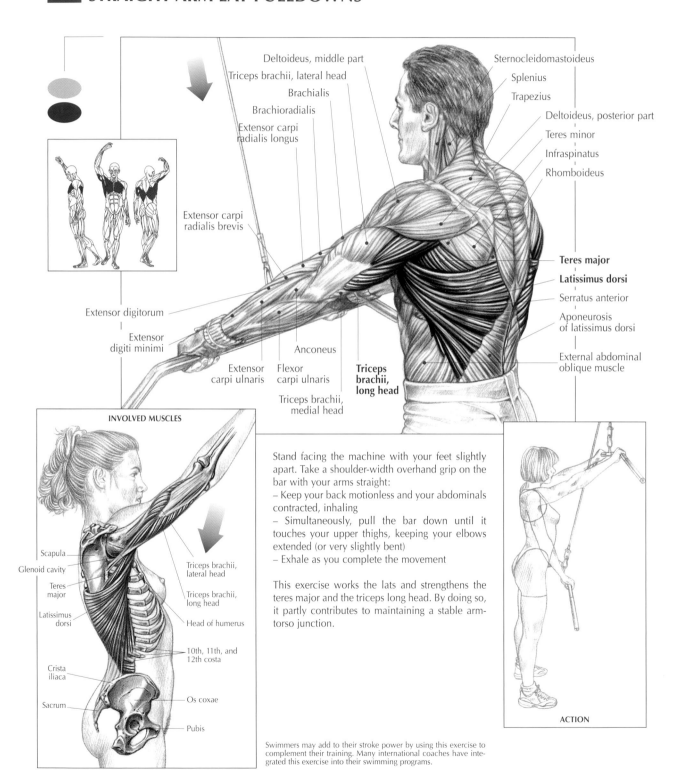

Deltoideus, middle part
Triceps brachii, lateral head
Brachialis
Brachioradialis
Extensor carpi radialis longus
Extensor carpi radialis brevis
Extensor digitorum
Extensor digiti minimi
Extensor carpi ulnaris
Flexor carpi ulnaris
Anconeus
Triceps brachii, medial head
Triceps brachii, long head

Sternocleidomastoideus
Splenius
Trapezius
Deltoideus, posterior part
Teres minor
Infraspinatus
Rhomboideus
Teres major
Latissimus dorsi
Serratus anterior
Aponeurosis of latissimus dorsi
External abdominal oblique muscle

INVOLVED MUSCLES

Scapula
Glenoid cavity
Teres major
Latissimus dorsi
Crista iliaca
Sacrum
Triceps brachii, lateral head
Triceps brachii, long head
Head of humerus
10th, 11th, and 12th costa
Os coxae
Pubis

Stand facing the machine with your feet slightly apart. Take a shoulder-width overhand grip on the bar with your arms straight:
– Keep your back motionless and your abdominals contracted, inhaling
– Simultaneously, pull the bar down until it touches your upper thighs, keeping your elbows extended (or very slightly bent)
– Exhale as you complete the movement

This exercise works the lats and strengthens the teres major and the triceps long head. By doing so, it partly contributes to maintaining a stable arm-torso junction.

ACTION

Swimmers may add to their stroke power by using this exercise to complement their training. Many international coaches have integrated this exercise into their swimming programs.

SEATED ROWS 7

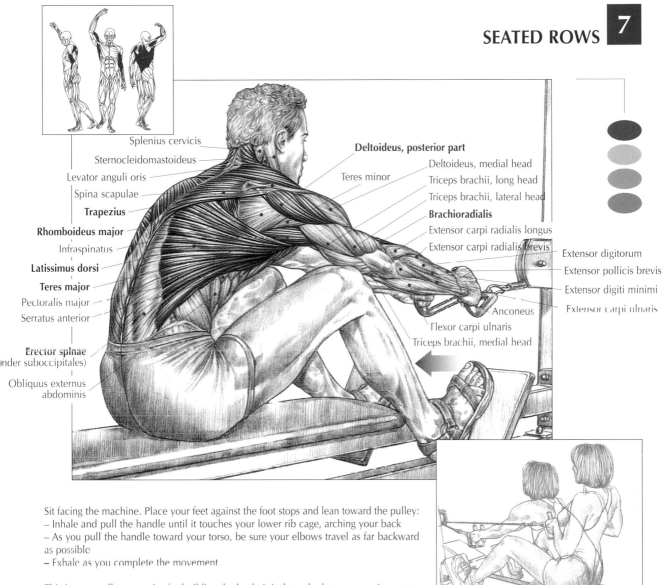

Splenius cervicis
Sternocleidomastoideus
Levator anguli oris
Spina scapulae
Trapezius
Rhomboideus major
Infraspinatus
Latissimus dorsi
Teres major
Pectoralis major
Serratus anterior
Erector spinae
(under suboccipitales)
Obliquus externus abdominis

Deltoideus, posterior part
Teres minor
Deltoideus, medial head
Triceps brachii, long head
Triceps brachii, lateral head
Brachioradialis
Extensor carpi radialis longus
Extensor carpi radialis brevis
Extensor digitorum
Extensor pollicis brevis
Extensor digiti minimi
Extensor carpi ulnaris
Anconeus
Flexor carpi ulnaris
Triceps brachii, medial head

Sit facing the machine. Place your feet against the foot stops and lean toward the pulley:
– Inhale and pull the handle until it touches your lower rib cage, arching your back
– As you pull the handle toward your torso, be sure your elbows travel as far backward as possible
– Exhale as you complete the movement

This is an excellent exercise for building the back. It isolates the lats, teres major, posterior deltoids, biceps, brachialis, brachioradialis, and, at the end of the movement when you press your scapulae together, the trapezius and rhomboid muscles. When you straighten, it also involves the spinal erectors. The negative phase of this movement, when you lean toward the pulley, completely stretches your lats.

Warning: to avoid the likelihood of back injury, never round your back as you do low pulley rows with heavy weight.

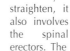

ACTION

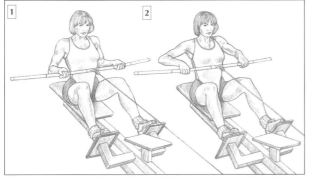

Straight-bar handle variation:
1. The underhand grip isolates the trapezius (lower portion), rhomboids, and biceps.
2. The overhand grip isolates the posterior deltoids and the middle portion of the trapezius.

8 ONE-ARM DUMBBELL ROWS

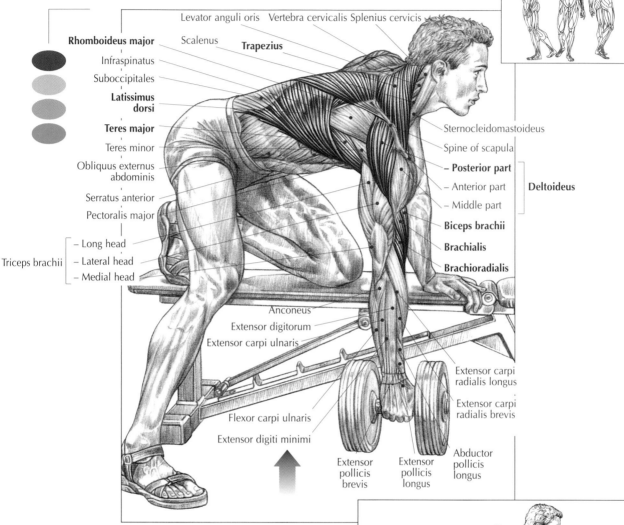

Levator anguli oris   Vertebra cervicalis   Splenius cervicis

Rhomboideus major   Scalenus   **Trapezius**

Infraspinatus

Suboccipitales

Latissimus dorsi

Teres major

Teres minor

Obliquus externus abdominis

Serratus anterior

Pectoralis major

Triceps brachii
– Long head
– Lateral head
– Medial head

Sternocleidomastoideus

Spine of scapula

– **Posterior part**

– Anterior part   **Deltoideus**

– Middle part

Biceps brachii

Brachialis

Brachioradialis

Anconeus

Extensor digitorum

Extensor carpi ulnaris

Flexor carpi ulnaris

Extensor digiti minimi

Extensor pollicis brevis

Extensor pollicis longus

Abductor pollicis longus

Extensor carpi radialis longus

Extensor carpi radialis brevis

Grasp the dumbbell with your palm facing in. Rest the opposite hand and knee on a bench:
– Steady your upper body in position, inhale and pull the dumbbell as high as possible, keeping your elbow back
– Be sure your upper arm travels a little away from your torso
– Exhale as you complete the movement

This exercise mainly works the lats, teres major, posterior deltoids, and the trapezius and rhomboid muscles at the end of the contraction. It places a secondary emphasis on the arm flexors, biceps, brachialis, and brachioradialis.

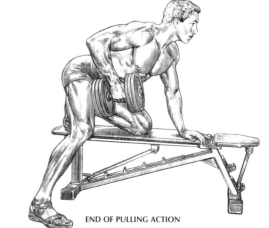

END OF PULLING ACTION

BENT ROWS 9

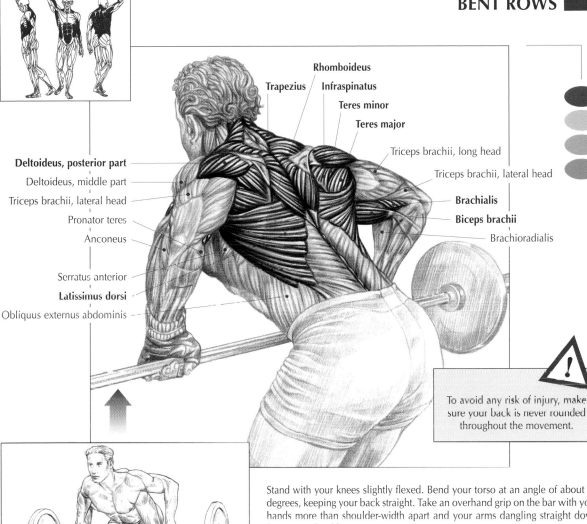

Rhomboideus

Trapezius   Infraspinatus

Teres minor

Teres major

Triceps brachii, long head

Triceps brachii, lateral head

Brachialis

Biceps brachii

Brachioradialis

Deltoideus, posterior part

Deltoideus, middle part

Triceps brachii, lateral head

Pronator teres

Anconeus

Serratus anterior

Latissimus dorsi

Obliquus externus abdominis

To avoid any risk of injury, make sure your back is never rounded throughout the movement.

ACTION

Stand with your knees slightly flexed. Bend your torso at an angle of about 45 degrees, keeping your back straight. Take an overhand grip on the bar with your hands more than shoulder-width apart and your arms dangling straight down from your shoulders:
– Inhale, contract your abdominals isometrically, and pull the bar straight up until it touches your chest:
– Return to the starting position, exhaling

This exercise works the lats, teres major, posterior deltoids, arm flexors, biceps, brachialis, brachioradialis, and, when you press your scapulae together at the end of the movement, the rhomboid and trapezius muscles.

Bending over works the spinal erectors isometrically.
You can work the back region at various angles by experimenting with different grip widths and types (overhand or underhand), as well as by varying the forward tilt of your torso.

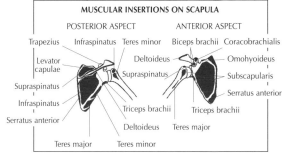

MUSCULAR INSERTIONS ON SCAPULA

POSTERIOR ASPECT   ANTERIOR ASPECT

Trapezius   Infraspinatus   Teres minor   Biceps brachii   Coracobrachialis

Levator capulae   Deltoideus   Omohyoideus

Supraspinatus   Supraspinatus   Subscapularis

Infraspinatus   Serratus anterior

Serratus anterior   Triceps brachii   Triceps brachii

Teres major   Deltoideus   Teres major

Teres major   Teres minor

10 T-BAR ROWS

Rhomboideus

Trapezius

Infraspinatus

Triceps brachii

Biceps brachii

Brachialis

Latissimus dorsi

Latissimus dorsi, aponeurosis of insertion

Obliquus externus abdominis

Splenius

Sternocleidomastoideus

Deltoideus, posterior part

Deltoideus, middle part

Brachioradialis

Extensor carpi radialis longus

Anconeus

Pectoralis minor

Pectoralis major

Serratus anterior

VARIATION WITH SPECIFIC MACHINE REPRODUCING T-BAR MOVEMENT

To avoid any risk of injury when doing T-bar rows without an incline bench, make sure your back is never rounded throughout the movement.

Back straight

Stand on the platforms provided on each side of the T-bar. Keep your knees slightly bent and your back straight. Bend over at about a 45-degree angle or rest against the incline bench if one is provided:
– Inhale and pull the T-bar up until the plates contact your chest
– Exhale as you complete the movement

This exercise, similar to bent rows, places more emphasis on the back and requires less effort to set your body in the correct movement pattern. It works the lats, teres major, posterior deltoids, arm flexors, and the trapezius and rhomboid muscles.

Note: if you take an underhand grip, you shift some work to the biceps and the upper portion of the trapezius at the end of the pull.

STIFF-LEGGED DEADLIFTS 11

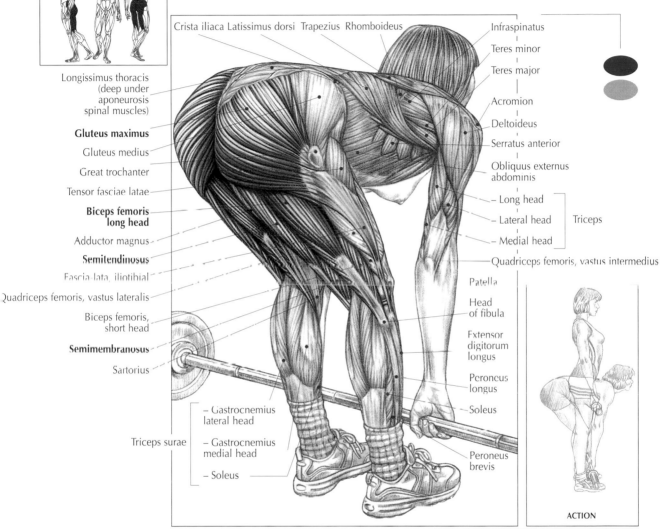

Crista iliaca Latissimus dorsi Trapezius Rhomboideus

Longissimus thoracis (deep under aponeurosis spinal muscles)

Gluteus maximus

Gluteus medius

Great trochanter

Tensor fasciae latae

Biceps femoris long head

Adductor magnus

Semitendinosus

Fascia lata, iliotibial

Quadriceps femoris, vastus lateralis

Biceps femoris, short head

Semimembranosus

Sartorius

– Gastrocnemius lateral head

– Gastrocnemius medial head

– Soleus

Triceps surae

Infraspinatus

Teres minor

Teres major

Acromion

Deltoideus

Serratus anterior

Obliquus externus abdominis

– Long head

– Lateral head   Triceps

– Medial head

Quadriceps femoris, vastus intermedius

Patella

Head of fibula

Extensor digitorum longus

Peroneus longus

Soleus

Peroneus brevis

ACTION

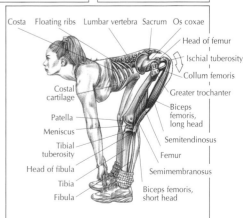

Costa Floating ribs Lumbar vertebra Sacrum Os coxae

Head of femur

Ischial tuberosity

Collum femoris

Greater trochanter

Biceps femoris, long head

Semitendinosus

Femur

Semimembranosus

Biceps femoris, short head

Costal cartilage

Patella

Meniscus

Tibial tuberosity

Head of fibula

Tibia

Fibula

Stand with your feet placed fairly close to each other, facing the bar on the floor. Bend forward at the waist, keeping your back arched and, if possible, your legs straight. Take an overhand grip on the bar, with your arms relaxed:
– Inhale and straighten your body, flexing at the hips and keeping your back rigid
– Exhale as you complete the movement and return the bar back to the floor, keeping your back straight

This exercise involves all the spinal erectors. When you flex at the hips to straighten your body, it specifically works the muscles of the hips, buttocks, and thighs (but not the thigh biceps short head).

The stiff-legged deadlift exercise stretches the back of your thighs. In order to increase the range of motion, perform the exercise while standing on a thick block of wood.

Warning: people with back problems should perform this exercise with caution because of the high amount of stress on the lumbar spine.

12 DEADLIFTS

Spinal cord
Processus spinosus
Nucleus pulposus
Processi articulares
Anulus fibrosus
Corpus vertebrae
Canalis vertebralis

When you flex your spine, the intervertebral disks are pinched at the front and gape at the back. The fluid of the nucleus pulposus moves backward and can compress nerve elements (which causes lumbago or sciatica).

Processus transversus
Processus articulares
Discus intervertebralis
Corpus vertebrae
Processus spinosus

Vertebral foramen (hole through which a nerve from the spinal cord runs).

Levator scapulae
Scalenus
Biceps brachii
Pectoralis major
Serratus anterior
Sternum
Brachialis

Sternocleido-mastoideus
Splenius cervicis
Trapezius
Deltoideus
Infraspinatus
Triceps brachii
Trapezius
Brachioradialis
Extensor carpi radialis longus
Anconeus
Extensor carpi radialis brevis
Extensor digitorum

Obliquus externus abdominalis
Rectus abdominis (under aponeurosis)
White line
Iliopsoas
Palmaris carpi longus
Flexor carpi radialis
Flexor digitorum

Extensor digiti minimi
Extensor carpi ulnaris
Flexor carpi ulnaris
Gluteus maximus
Iliotibial tract, fascia lata

Pectineus
Adductor longus
Adductor magnus
Gracilis
Sartorius
Patella

– Rectus femoris
– Vastus lateralis
– Vastus medialis
– Biceps femoris

Quadriceps

Triceps surae
– Gastrocnemius, lateral head
– Gastrocnemius, medial head
– Soleus
Tibia, medial side
Flexor digitorum longus

Tibialis anterior
Peroneus longus
Extensor digitorum longus
Peroneus brevis

Stand facing the bar with your feet slightly spread. Keep your back motionless and a little arched. Flex your knees until your thighs are almost parallel to the floor. Depending on your physique and the flexibility of your ankles, you can vary this position (for example, if your thigh bones and arms are short, place your thighs in a horizontal position ; if your thigh bones and arms are long, place your thighs a little above your knees). Take an overhand grip on the bar, with your hands slightly more than shoulder-width apart (you can also use an over-under grip (one palm faces forward and the other faces back) to prevent the bar from rolling and to work with much heavier weight):
– Inhale, contract your abdominal and low back muscles, and lift the bar by straightening your legs (contracting your abdominals and keeping your back straight), raising it in front of your shins
– When the bar reaches your knees, extend your torso so you are standing erect with your arms straight down at your sides, exhaling as you complete the movement
– Hold this straightened position for 2 seconds, then return the weight to the floor, making sure you do not hyperextend or arch your back

This exercise works virtually every muscle. It builds terrific hip, lower back, and trapezius muscle mass. It also involves the buttocks and quadriceps. With the bench press and the squat, it is one of the movements performed in powerlifting events.

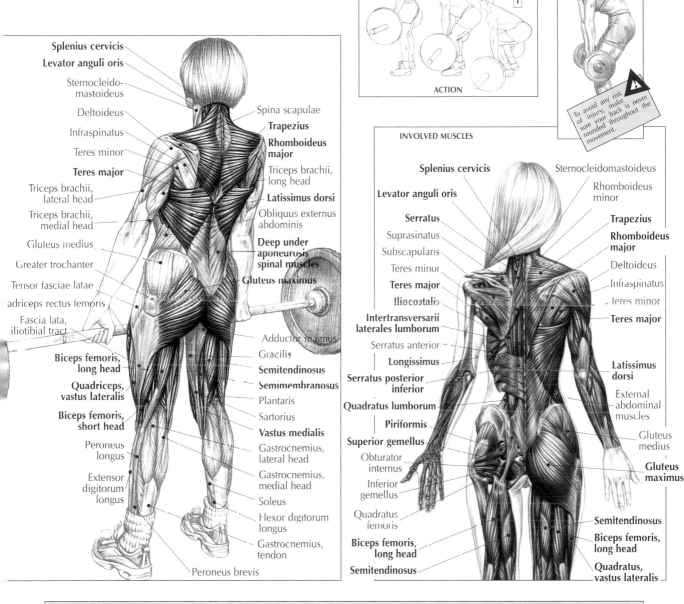

ACTION

To avoid any risk of injury, make sure your back is never rounded throughout the movement.

INVOLVED MUSCLES

Splenius cervicis
Levator anguli oris
Sternocleido-
mastoideus
Deltoideus
Infraspinatus
Teres minor
Teres major
Triceps brachii,
lateral head
Triceps brachii,
medial head
Gluteus medius
Greater trochanter
Tensor fasciae latae
adriceps rectus femoris
Fascia lata,
iliotibial tract
**Biceps femoris,
long head**
**Quadriceps,
vastus lateralis**
**Biceps femoris,
short head**
Peroneus
longus
Extensor
digitorum
longus

Spina scapulae
Trapezius
**Rhomboideus
major**
Triceps brachii,
long head
Latissimus dorsi
Obliquus externus
abdominis
**Deep under
aponeurosis
spinal muscles**
Gluteus maximus
Adductor magnus
Gracilis
Semitendinosus
Semimembranosus
Plantaris
Sartorius
Vastus medialis
Gastrocnemius,
lateral head
Gastrocnemius,
medial head
Soleus
Flexor digitorum
longus
Gastrocnemius,
tendon
Peroneus brevis

Splenius cervicis
Levator anguli oris
Serratus
Suprasinatus
Subscapularis
Teres minor
Teres major
Iliocostalis
**Intertransversarii
laterales lumborum**
Serratus anterior
Longissimus
**Serratus posterior
inferior**
Quadratus lumborum
Piriformis
Superior gemellus
Obturator
internus
Inferior
gemellus
Quadratus
femoris
**Biceps femoris,
long head**
Semitendinosus

Sternocleidomastoideus
Rhomboideus
minor
Trapezius
**Rhomboideus
major**
Deltoideus
Infraspinatus
Teres minor
Teres major
**Latissimus
dorsi**
External
abdominal
muscles
Gluteus
medius
**Gluteus
maximus**
Semitendinosus
**Biceps femoris,
long head**
**Quadratus,
vastus lateralis**

In any movement, whenever you use heavy weight, you must "**block**."
1. Stick out your chest by taking a deep breath and filling your lungs with air like a balloon. In this way, you will stiffen your rib cage and prevent your upper torso from bending forward.
2. Contract all the abdominal muscles to increase intra-abdominal pressure so your shoulders are pulled back when you are in the top position of the movement.
3. Finally, contract the lower back muscles to arch your lower back and extend the bottom of the spine.
These three simultaneous actions are called "**blocking**." Their function is to avoid rounding the back (or flexing the spine), which may cause a slipped disk if you work with heavy weight.

13 SUMO DEADLIFTS

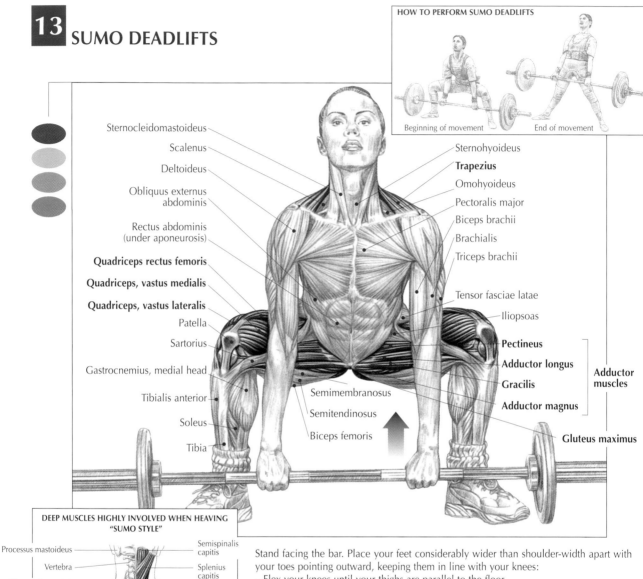

HOW TO PERFORM SUMO DEADLIFTS

Beginning of movement   End of movement

Sternocleidomastoideus
Scalenus
Deltoideus
Obliquus externus abdominis
Rectus abdominis (under aponeurosis)
Quadriceps rectus femoris
Quadriceps, vastus medialis
Quadriceps, vastus lateralis
Patella
Sartorius
Gastrocnemius, medial head
Tibialis anterior
Soleus
Tibia

Sternohyoideus
Trapezius
Omohyoideus
Pectoralis major
Biceps brachii
Brachialis
Triceps brachii
Tensor fasciae latae
Iliopsoas
Pectineus
Adductor longus
Gracilis
Adductor magnus
Adductor muscles
Gluteus maximus

Semimembranosus
Semitendinosus
Biceps femoris

DEEP MUSCLES HIGHLY INVOLVED WHEN HEAVING "SUMO STYLE"

Processus mastoideus
Vertebra
Iliocostalis cervicis
Longissimus cervicis
Costa
Iliocostalis thoracis
Longissimus thoracis
Intertransversarii laterales lumborum
Iliocostalis lumborum
Quadratus lumborum
Aponeurosis of insertion

Semispinalis capitis
Splenius capitis
Splenius cervicis
Serratus, posterior superior
Serratus posterior inferior
Os coxae
Sacrum
Coccyx
Femur

Stand facing the bar. Place your feet considerably wider than shoulder-width apart with your toes pointing outward, keeping them in line with your knees:
– Flex your knees until your thighs are parallel to the floor
– Take an overhand grip on the bar with your hands about shoulder-width apart, keeping your arms straight (use an over-under grip to lift heavier loads)
– Inhale, hold your breath, slightly arch your back, shoulders backward, contract your abdominals and straighten your legs, extending your torso to stand erect. Exhale.

Unlike normal deadlifts, this exercise places primary emphasis on the quadriceps and adductors and secondary emphasis on the back, because it is not as much bend as at the beginning.

When you lift heavy weight, be sure to do this movement very carefully; execute the proper technique to avoid traumatizing the hips and the adductors of the thighs, as well as the connection between the sacrum and the lumbar vertebrae, which is directly involved in the exercise.

The sumo deadlift is one of the three powerlifting movements.

Note: at the beginning of the movement, make sure you raise the bar in front of your tibias. At the end of the movement, keep your back straight, holding your breath.

BACK EXTENSION

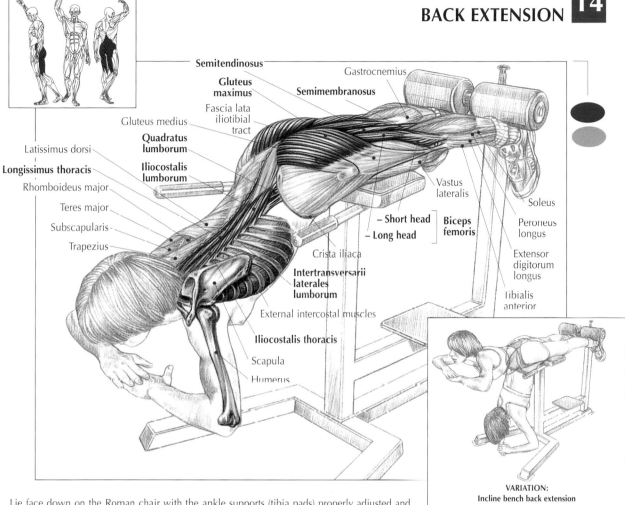

Semitendinosus
Gluteus maximus
Semimembranosus
Gastrocnemius
Fascia lata iliotibial tract
Gluteus medius
Quadratus lumborum
Latissimus dorsi
Longissimus thoracis
Iliocostalis lumborum
Rhomboideus major
Vastus lateralis
Teres major
– Short head
– Long head
Biceps femoris
Subscapularis
Soleus
Trapezius
Peroneus longus
Crista iliaca
Extensor digitorum longus
Intertransversarii laterales lumborum
Tibialis anterior
External intercostal muscles
Iliocostalis thoracis
Scapula
Humerus

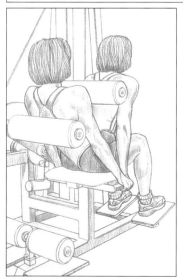

VARIATION:
Incline bench back extension

Lie face down on the Roman chair with the ankle supports (tibia pads) properly adjusted and your hips on the support pads:
– Start with your thighs flexed and raise your upper body to a position parallel to the floor
– Be sure to assume the proper arched position to reduce the chance of injury to the lower back

This exercise places primary emphasis on the buttocks and thigh biceps (except the thigh biceps short head) and secondary emphasis on the spinal erectors and other lower back muscles. In addition, flexing the upper body completely is excellent for stretching all the sacrospinalis muscles. Placing your pelvis on the front padded surface moves the axis of flexion forward and isolates the work on the sacrospinalis, but with less intensity because of the limited range of movement and increased leverage.

You can hold the hyperextension for a few seconds to help isolate the work.
Beginners can perform this exercise on a specific incline bench for more comfort.

Variation: with a specific machine, you can isolate the stress on the sacrospinalis.

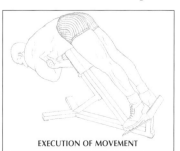

EXECUTION OF MOVEMENT

15 UPRIGHT ROWS

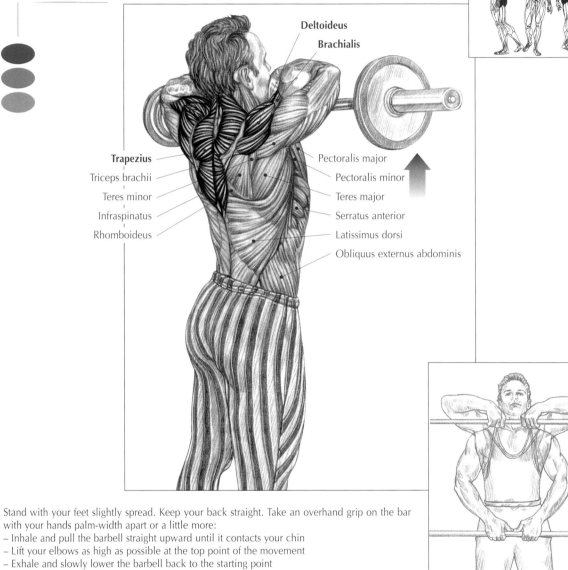

Deltoideus

Brachialis

Trapezius

Triceps brachii

Teres minor

Infraspinatus

Rhomboideus

Pectoralis major

Pectoralis minor

Teres major

Serratus anterior

Latissimus dorsi

Obliquus externus abdominis

ACTION

Stand with your feet slightly spread. Keep your back straight. Take an overhand grip on the bar with your hands palm-width apart or a little more:
– Inhale and pull the barbell straight upward until it contacts your chin
– Lift your elbows as high as possible at the top point of the movement
– Exhale and slowly lower the barbell back to the starting point

This exercise works the upper trapezius and medial-posterior deltoid groups most intensely. Secondary emphasis is placed on the anterior deltoids, biceps, forearm flexors, abdominals, buttocks, and sacrospinalis.
The wider your grip, the more the movement works the deltoids and the less it works the trapezius muscles.

BARBELL SHRUGS 16

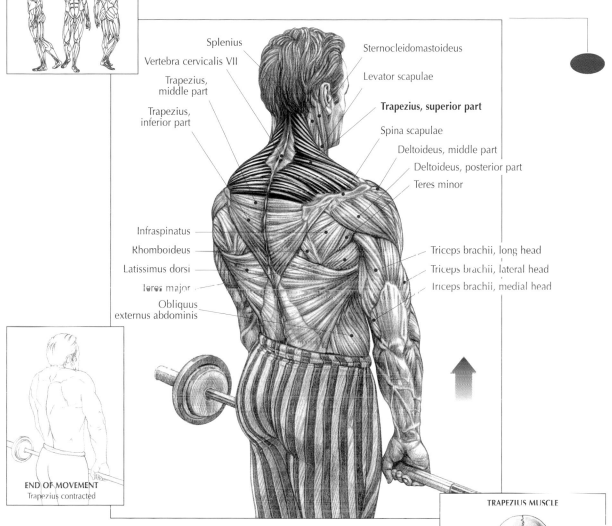

Splenius
Vertebra cervicalis VII
Trapezius, middle part
Trapezius, inferior part

Sternocleidomastoideus
Levator scapulae
Trapezius, superior part
Spina scapulae
Deltoideus, middle part
Deltoideus, posterior part
Teres minor

Infraspinatus
Rhomboideus
Latissimus dorsi
Teres major
Obliquus externus abdominis

Triceps brachii, long head
Triceps brachii, lateral head
Triceps brachii, medial head

END OF MOVEMENT
Trapezius contracted

TRAPEZIUS MUSCLE

Cranium
Spina scapulae
Trapezius

Linea nuchae superior
Clavicula
Acromion

Scapula

Costa

Thoracic vertebra

Stand with your feet slightly apart, facing the bar resting on the floor or on a weight rack:
– Take an overhand grip on the bar (or an over-under grip if the weight is heavy), with your hands a little more than shoulder-width apart
– Keeping your arms and back straight, contract your abdominals and shrug your shoulders upward and to the rear as high as possible

This exercise isolates the trapezius muscles. Secondary emphasis is placed on the deltoids.

17 DUMBBELL SHRUGS

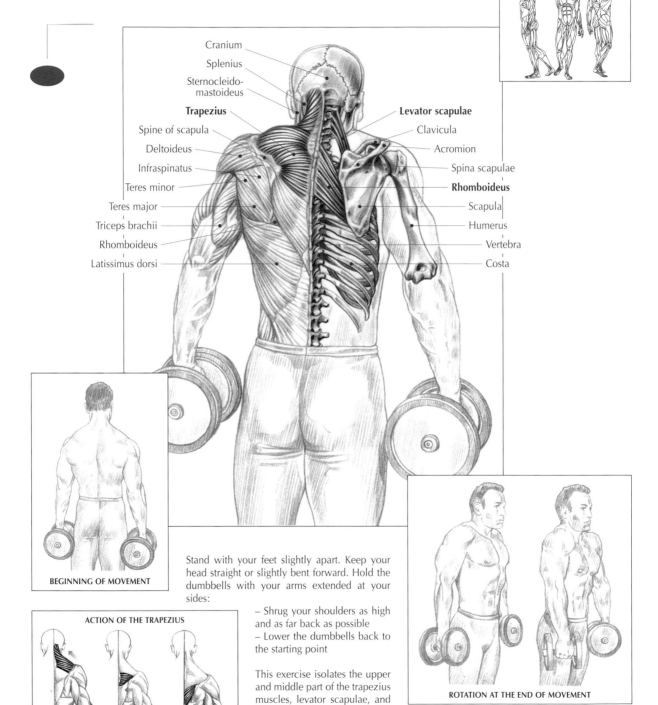

Cranium
Splenius
Sternocleido-mastoideus
Trapezius
Spine of scapula
Deltoideus
Infraspinatus
Teres minor
Teres major
Triceps brachii
Rhomboideus
Latissimus dorsi

Levator scapulae
Clavicula
Acromion
Spina scapulae
Rhomboideus
Scapula
Humerus
Vertebra
Costa

BEGINNING OF MOVEMENT

ACTION OF THE TRAPEZIUS

Stand with your feet slightly apart. Keep your head straight or slightly bent forward. Hold the dumbbells with your arms extended at your sides:

– Shrug your shoulders as high and as far back as possible
– Lower the dumbbells back to the starting point

This exercise isolates the upper and middle part of the trapezius muscles, levator scapulae, and the rhomboids when you press your scapulae together to shrug your shoulders to the rear.

ROTATION AT THE END OF MOVEMENT

MACHINE SHRUGS 18

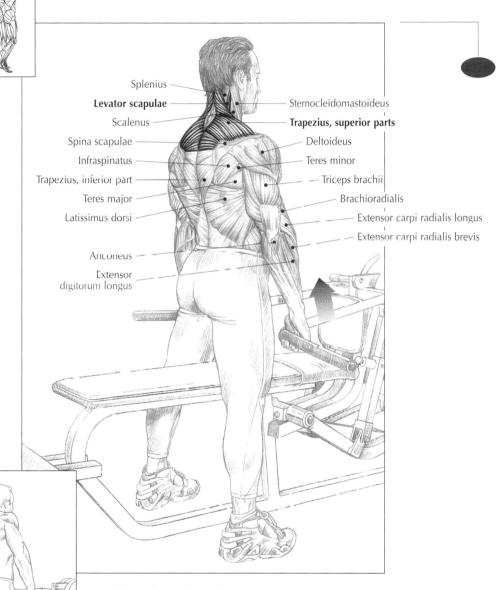

Splenius
Levator scapulae
Scalenus
Spina scapulae
Infraspinatus
Trapezius, inferior part
Teres major
Latissimus dorsi

Anconeus
Extensor digitorum longus

Sternocleidomastoideus
Trapezius, superior parts
Deltoideus
Teres minor
Triceps brachii
Brachioradialis
Extensor carpi radialis longus
Extensor carpi radialis brevis

END OF MOVEMENT
Trapezius contracted

Stand facing the machine. Take an overhand grip on the bar, with your hands slightly more than shoulder-width apart or, if the machine allows it, with your palms facing each other:
– Keep your head and back straight and shrug your shoulders
– Return to the starting position

This exercise is excellent for developing the upper part of the trapezius and the levator scapulae.

5 LEGS

1. Dumbbell Squats
2. Squats
3. Front Squats
4. Power Squats
5. Angled Leg Press
6. Hack Squats
7. Leg Extensions
8. Lying Leg Curls
9. Standing Leg Curls
10. Seated Leg Curls
11. Good Mornings
12. Cable Adductions
13. Machine Adductions
14. Standing Calf Raises
15. One-Leg Toe Raises
16. Donkey Calf Raises
17. Seated Calf Raises
18. Seated Barbell Calf Raises

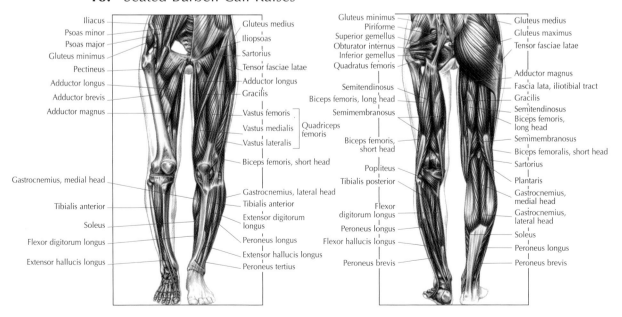

DUMBBELL SQUATS

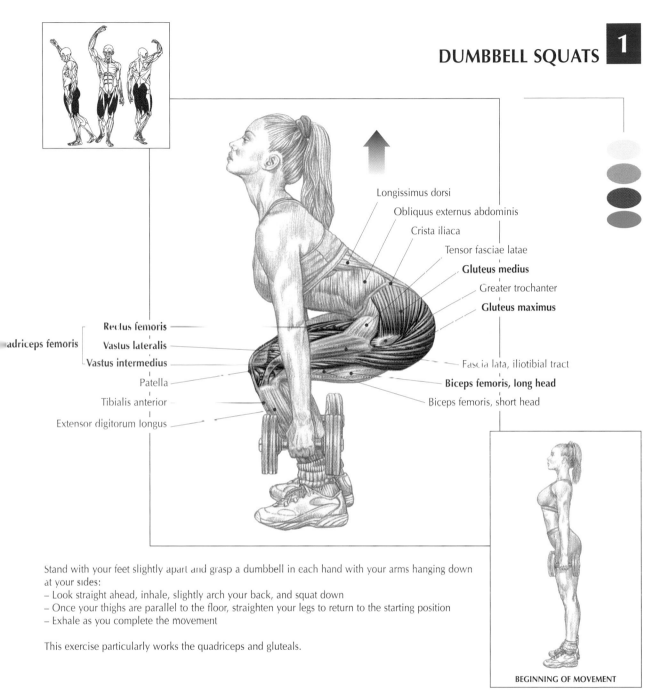

Longissimus dorsi
Obliquus externus abdominis
Crista iliaca
Tensor fasciae latae
Gluteus medius
Greater trochanter
Gluteus maximus

Fascia lata, iliotibial tract
Biceps femoris, long head
Biceps femoris, short head

adriceps femoris

Rectus femoris
Vastus lateralis
Vastus intermedius
Patella
Tibialis anterior
Extensor digitorum longus

BEGINNING OF MOVEMENT

Stand with your feet slightly apart and grasp a dumbbell in each hand with your arms hanging down at your sides:
– Look straight ahead, inhale, slightly arch your back, and squat down
– Once your thighs are parallel to the floor, straighten your legs to return to the starting position
– Exhale as you complete the movement

This exercise particularly works the quadriceps and gluteals.

2 SQUATS

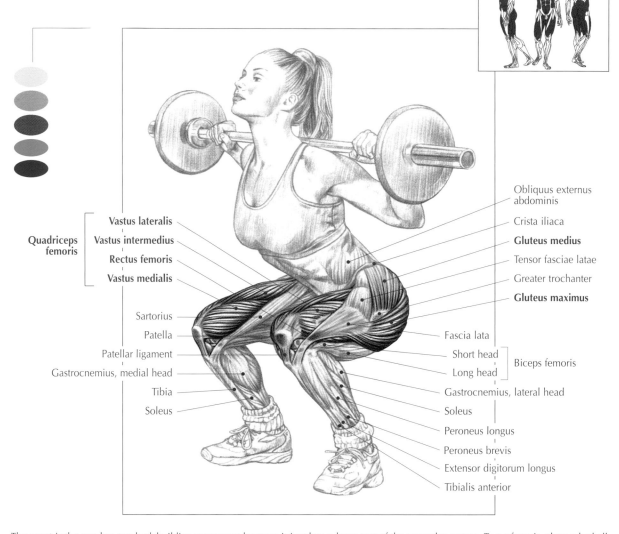

Quadriceps femoris
- **Vastus lateralis**
- **Vastus intermedius**
- **Rectus femoris**
- **Vastus medialis**

Sartorius
Patella
Patellar ligament
Gastrocnemius, medial head
Tibia
Soleus

Obliquus externus abdominis
Crista iliaca
Gluteus medius
Tensor fasciae latae
Greater trochanter
Gluteus maximus

Fascia lata
Short head } Biceps femoris
Long head
Gastrocnemius, lateral head
Soleus
Peroneus longus
Peroneus brevis
Extensor digitorum longus
Tibialis anterior

The squat is the number one bodybuilding movement because it involves a large part of the muscular system. To perform it, place a barbell on a squat rack. Duck under the bar and position it across your shoulders on the trapezius, slighly above the posterior part of the deltoids. Grasp the bar using a grip width appropriate to your body type and pull your elbows to the rear:

– Inhale deeply (to maintain intrathoracic pressure and prevent your-self from bending forward) and slightly arch your back by rotating your pelvis forward
– Look straight ahead and lift the bar off the rack
– Move back a step or two from the rack and set your feet shoulder-width apart, keeping your toes pointed forward or slightly angled outward
– Slowly bend your knees and squat down your back slightly bent forward

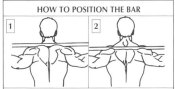

HOW TO POSITION THE BAR

1. On the trapezius
2. On the trapezius and deltoids posterior part, as in the type of squat powerlifters do in competition

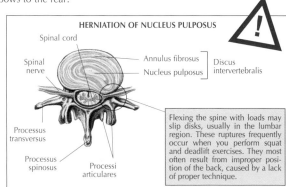

HERNIATION OF NUCLEUS PULPOSUS

Spinal cord
Spinal nerve
Annulus fibrosus } Discus intervertebralis
Nucleus pulposus
Processus transversus
Processus spinosus
Processi articulares

Flexing the spine with loads may slip disks, usually in the lumbar region. These ruptures frequently occur when you perform squat and deadlift exercises. They most often result from improper posi-tion of the back, caused by a lack of proper technique.

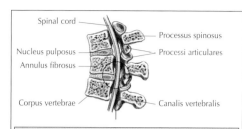

When you flex your spine, the intervertebral disks are pinched at the front and gape at the back. The fluid of the nucleus pulposus moves backward and can compress nerve elements (which causes lumbago or sciatica).

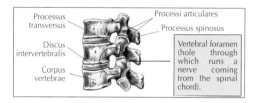

– To avoid injury, keep your back straight (the axis of flexion runs through the hip-thigh joint)
– Once your thighs are parallel to the floor, extend your legs and straighten your torso to return to the starting (upright) position
– Exhale as you complete the movement

Squats particularly work the quadriceps, gluteals, adductors, spinal erectors, abdominals, and hamstrings.

Variations:

(1) If you have inflexible ankles or long thigh bones, rest your heels on a block of wood to avoid bending too far forward. This variation shifts part of the stress to the quadriceps. However, this variation can position the knees too far forward for safe lifting so use it with caution.
(2) You can position the bar lower, across your upper deltoids, to improve your balance and increase the lifting power of your back, which allows you to use heavier weight. This technique is mostly used by powerlifters.
(3) You can do squats on a specific machine to prevent yourself from bending forward and isolate stress on the quadriceps.

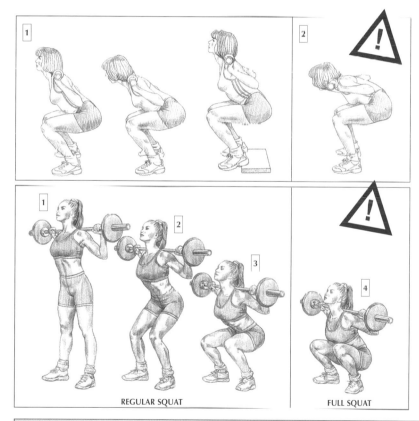

REGULAR SQUAT

FULL SQUAT

1. PROPER POSITIONS:
When doing squats, always keep your back as upright as possible.
There are differences in body types (legs of different lengths, ankles more or less flexible) and different ways to execute the technique (experimenting with different foot-stance widths, using platform shoes or heelpieces, resting the barbell higher or lower on the traps). Consequently, your torso will be more or less inclined, but be sure to bend forward at thight joint.

2. IMPROPER POSITION:
Never flex the spine while doing squats. This error contributes to most low back injuries, especially slipped disks.

In order to correctly feel the action of the gluteals, it is important to bend your knees until your thighs are parallel to the floor.

1–3: NEGATIVE PHASE OF REGULAR SQUAT

4. FULL SQUAT:
To place more emphasis on the gluteals, you can bring your thighs into a position below the horizontal. However, use this technique only if you have flexible ankles or short thigh bones. In addition, do the full squat carefully because it tends to flex the spine, which can lead to serious injuries.

In any movement, whenever you use heavy weight, you must "**block**."
1. Stick out your chest by taking a deep breath and filling your lungs with air like a balloon. In this way, you will stiffen your rib cage and prevent your upper torso from bending forward.
2. Contract all the abdominal muscles to increase intra-abdominal pressure so your shoulders are pulled back when you are in the top position of the movement.
3. Finally, contract the lower back muscles to arch your lower back and extend the bottom of the spine.
These three simultaneous actions are called "**blocking**." Their function is to avoid rounding the back (or flexing the spine), which will cause a slipped disk if you work with heavy weight.

3 FRONT SQUATS

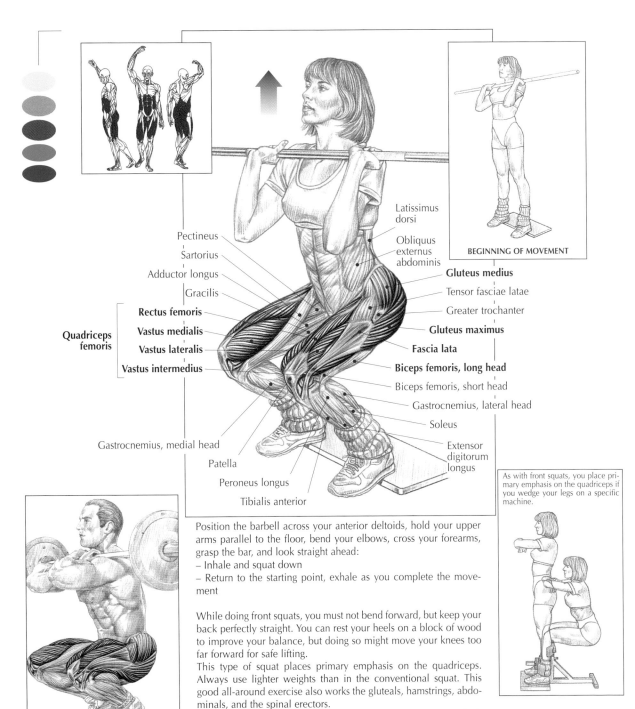

BEGINNING OF MOVEMENT

Latissimus dorsi

Obliquus externus abdominis

Gluteus medius

Tensor fasciae latae

Greater trochanter

Gluteus maximus

Fascia lata

Biceps femoris, long head

Biceps femoris, short head

Gastrocnemius, lateral head

Soleus

Extensor digitorum longus

Pectineus

Sartorius

Adductor longus

Gracilis

Rectus femoris

Quadriceps femoris

Vastus medialis

Vastus lateralis

Vastus intermedius

Gastrocnemius, medial head

Patella

Peroneus longus

Tibialis anterior

CROSSED ARMS VARIATION

As with front squats, you place primary emphasis on the quadriceps if you wedge your legs on a specific machine.

Position the barbell across your anterior deltoids, hold your upper arms parallel to the floor, bend your elbows, cross your forearms, grasp the bar, and look straight ahead:
– Inhale and squat down
– Return to the starting point, exhale as you complete the movement

While doing front squats, you must not bend forward, but keep your back perfectly straight. You can rest your heels on a block of wood to improve your balance, but doing so might move your knees too far forward for safe lifting.

This type of squat places primary emphasis on the quadriceps. Always use lighter weights than in the conventional squat. This good all-around exercise also works the gluteals, hamstrings, abdominals, and the spinal erectors.

Weightlifters often use this movement because it works the thigh muscles exactly the same way as when doing cleans or finishing snatches.

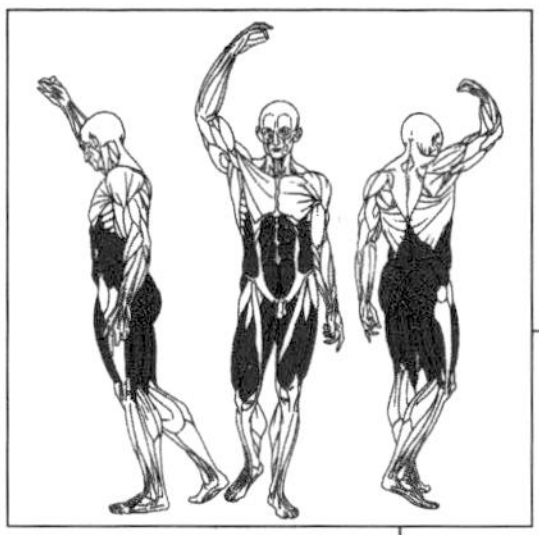

POWER SQUATS 4

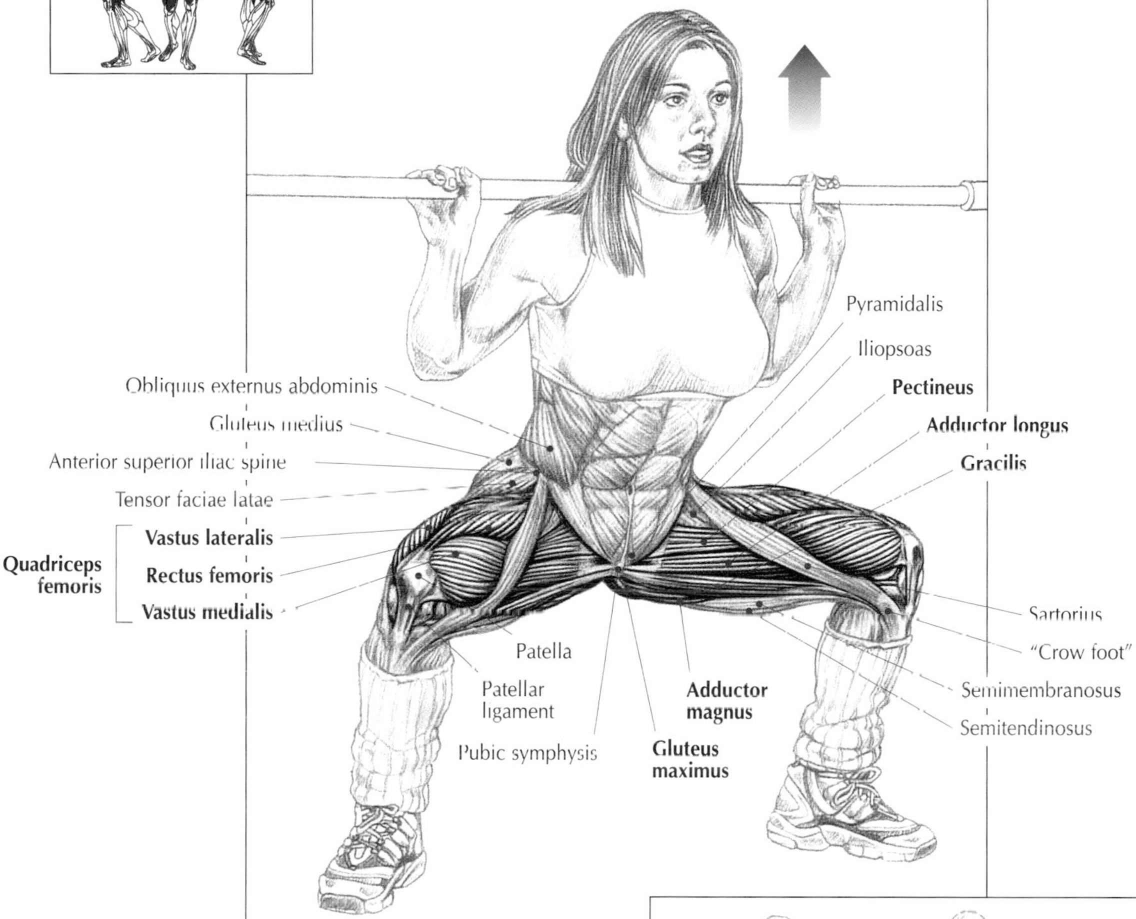

Pyramidalis

Iliopsoas

Pectineus

Adductor longus

Gracilis

Obliquus externus abdominis

Gluteus medius

Anterior superior iliac spine

Tensor faciae latae

Vastus lateralis

Quadriceps femoris **Rectus femoris**

Vastus medialis

Sartorius

"Crow foot"

Semimembranosus

Semitendinosus

Patella

Patellar ligament

Pubic symphysis

Adductor magnus

Gluteus maximus

This movement is the same as conventional squats, but your legs are widely spread with your toes pointed outward, which specifically works the inner thighs.

The muscles involved are
– the quadriceps,
– all the adductors (adductor longus, adductor magnus, adductor brevis, pectineus and gracilis),
– the gluteals,
– the hamstring group, and
– all the sacrospinalis muscles.

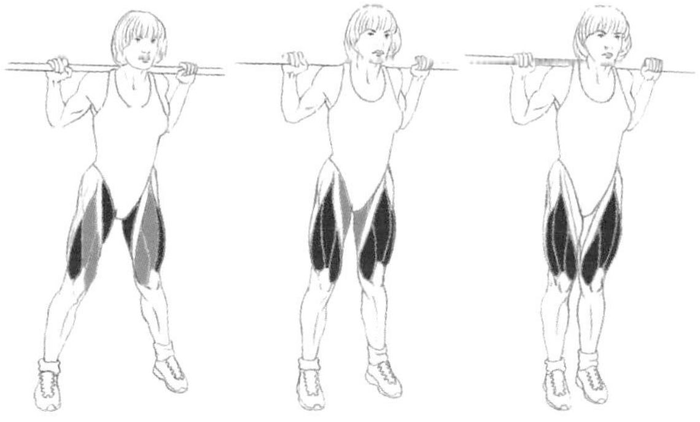

THE THREE FOOT STANCES TO DO SQUATS

More involved muscles   Involved muscles

5 ANGLED LEG PRESS

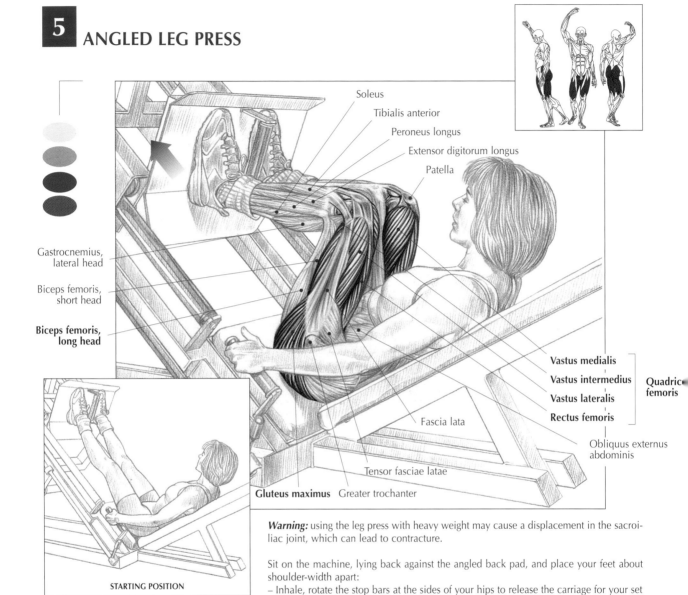

Soleus
Tibialis anterior
Peroneus longus
Extensor digitorum longus
Patella

Gastrocnemius, lateral head

Biceps femoris, short head

Biceps femoris, long head

Vastus medialis
Vastus intermedius } Quadriceps femoris
Vastus lateralis
Rectus femoris

Fascia lata

Obliquus externus abdominis

Tensor fasciae latae

Gluteus maximus Greater trochanter

STARTING POSITION

Warning: using the leg press with heavy weight may cause a displacement in the sacroiliac joint, which can lead to contracture.

Sit on the machine, lying back against the angled back pad, and place your feet about shoulder-width apart:
– Inhale, rotate the stop bars at the sides of your hips to release the carriage for your set
– Bend your legs as much as possible while making sure your knees travel to the sides of your chest
– Return to the starting position, exhaling as you complete the movement

If you place your feet lower on the footplate, you will primarily stress your quadriceps. Conversely, if you place your feet on the top of the footplate, you will shift more emphasis to the buttocks and hamstrings. If you spread your legs, the adductors will be more involved. If you have back problems, you can do this movement instead of squats. However, always keep your buttocks on the pad.

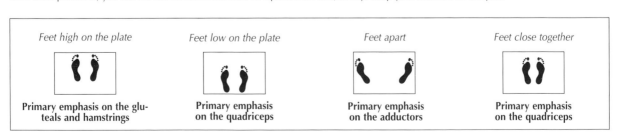

Feet high on the plate

Primary emphasis on the gluteals and hamstrings

Feet low on the plate

Primary emphasis on the quadriceps

Feet apart

Primary emphasis on the adductors

Feet close together

Primary emphasis on the quadriceps

HACK SQUATS 6

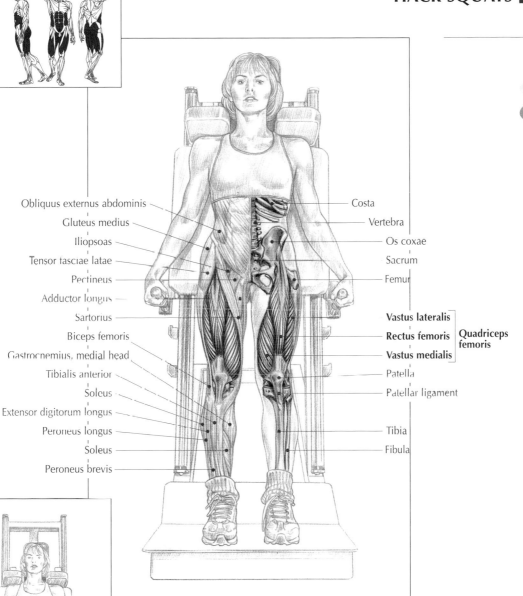

Obliquus externus abdominis
Gluteus medius
Iliopsoas
Tensor fasciae latae
Pectineus
Adductor longus
Sartorius
Biceps femoris
Gastrocnemius, medial head
Tibialis anterior
Soleus
Extensor digitorum longus
Peroneus longus
Soleus
Peroneus brevis

Costa
Vertebra
Os coxae
Sacrum
Femur
Vastus lateralis
Rectus femoris Quadriceps femoris
Vastus medialis
Patella
Patellar ligament
Tibia
Fibula

Flex your knees, place your back against the padded surface, wedge your shoulders beneath the yokes attached to the machine, and place your feet fairly close together:
– Inhale, rotate the stop handles at the sides of the yokes to release the machine, and bend your legs
– Return to the starting position, exhaling as you complete the movement

This movement maximizes emphasis on the quadriceps. If you place your feet close together, you will place more emphasis on the gluteals. If you spread your feet, you will shift the work to the adductors. To protect your back from injury, be sure to contract your abdominals in order to avoid swinging your pelvis and spine.

7 LEG EXTENSIONS

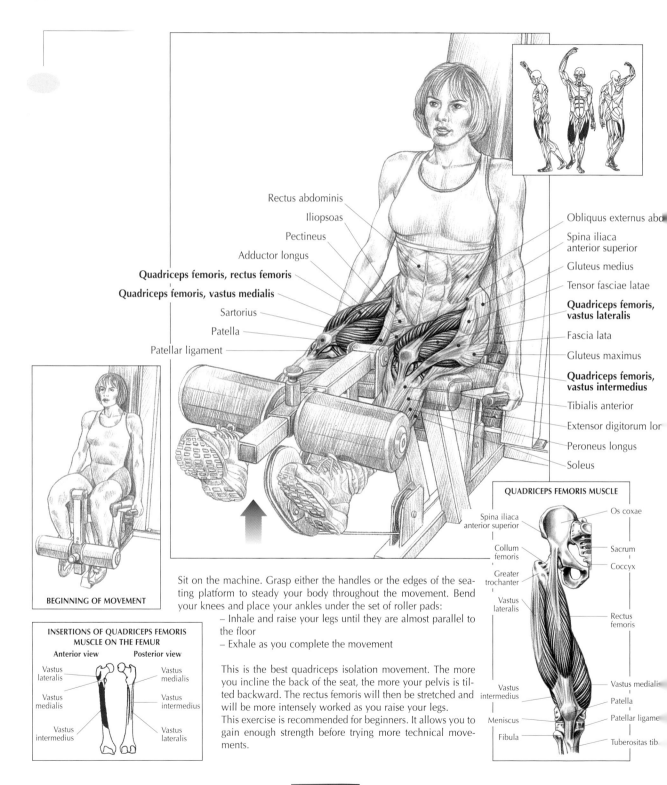

Rectus abdominis

Iliopsoas

Pectineus

Adductor longus

Quadriceps femoris, rectus femoris

Quadriceps femoris, vastus medialis

Sartorius

Patella

Patellar ligament

Obliquus externus abd

Spina iliaca
anterior superior

Gluteus medius

Tensor fasciae latae

**Quadriceps femoris,
vastus lateralis**

Fascia lata

Gluteus maximus

**Quadriceps femoris,
vastus intermedius**

Tibialis anterior

Extensor digitorum lor

Peroneus longus

Soleus

BEGINNING OF MOVEMENT

QUADRICEPS FEMORIS MUSCLE

Spina iliaca
anterior superior

Os coxae

Collum
femoris

Sacrum

Greater
trochanter

Coccyx

Vastus
lateralis

Rectus
femoris

Vastus
intermedius

Vastus medialis

Patella

Meniscus

Patellar ligame

Fibula

Tuberositas tib

**INSERTIONS OF QUADRICEPS FEMORIS
MUSCLE ON THE FEMUR**

Anterior view   **Posterior view**

Vastus
lateralis

Vastus
medialis

Vastus
medialis

Vastus
intermedius

Vastus
intermedius

Vastus
lateralis

Sit on the machine. Grasp either the handles or the edges of the sea-
ting platform to steady your body throughout the movement. Bend
your knees and place your ankles under the set of roller pads:
— Inhale and raise your legs until they are almost parallel to
the floor
— Exhale as you complete the movement

This is the best quadriceps isolation movement. The more
you incline the back of the seat, the more your pelvis is til-
ted backward. The rectus femoris will then be stretched and
will be more intensely worked as you raise your legs.
This exercise is recommended for beginners. It allows you to
gain enough strength before trying more technical movements.

LYING LEG CURLS **8**

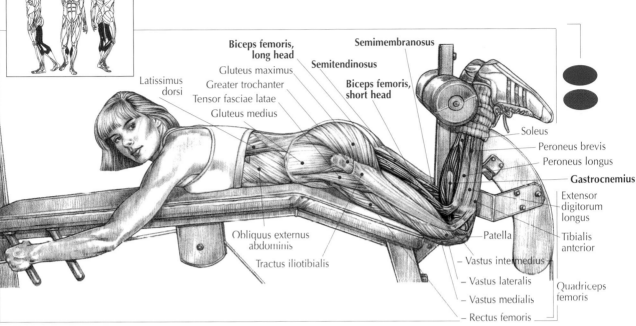

Biceps femoris, long head
Semimembranosus
Semitendinosus
Biceps femoris, short head
Latissimus dorsi
Gluteus maximus
Greater trochanter
Tensor fasciae latae
Gluteus medius
Soleus
Peroneus brevis
Peroneus longus
Gastrocnemius
Extensor digitorum longus
Tibialis anterior
Patella
Obliquus externus abdominis
Tractus iliotibialis
Vastus intermedius
Vastus lateralis
Vastus medialis
Rectus femoris
Quadriceps femoris

Lie facedown on the padded surface of the machine. Grasp the handles, straighten your knees and hook your feet under the set of roller pads:
– Inhale and simultaneously raise your feet upward until your knees are as fully bent as possible (try to touch your buttocks with your heels)
– Exhale as you complete the movement
– Slowly return to the starting position

This exercise involves the entire hamstring group as well as the gastrocnemius. In theory, as you curl your feet upward you can place more emphasis on either the semitendinosus and semimembranosus (by angling your toes inward) or on the biceps femoris long and short heads (by angling your toes outward). However, in practice it turns out to be difficult, and only the placing of primary emphasis on the hamstrings or gastrocnemius is easy:
– feet extended puts more stress on the hamstrings
– feet dorsiflexed puts more stress on the gastrocnemius

Variation: you can perform this exercise with one leg at a time or by holding a barbell with both feet.

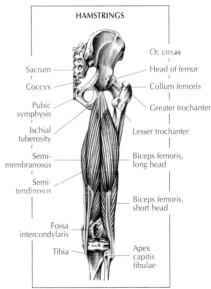

HAMSTRINGS

Sacrum
Coccyx
Pubic symphysis
Ischial tuberosity
Semi-membranosus
Semi-tendinosus
Fossa intercondylaris
Tibia
Os coxae
Head of femur
Collum femoris
Greater trochanter
Lesser trochanter
Biceps femoris, long head
Biceps femoris, short head
Apex capitis fibulae

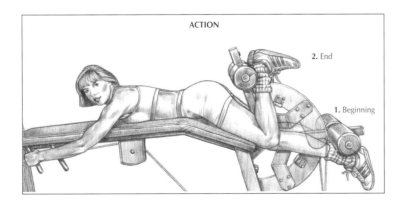

ACTION

2. End

1. Beginning

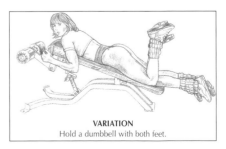

VARIATION
Hold a dumbbell with both feet.

9 STANDING LEG CURLS

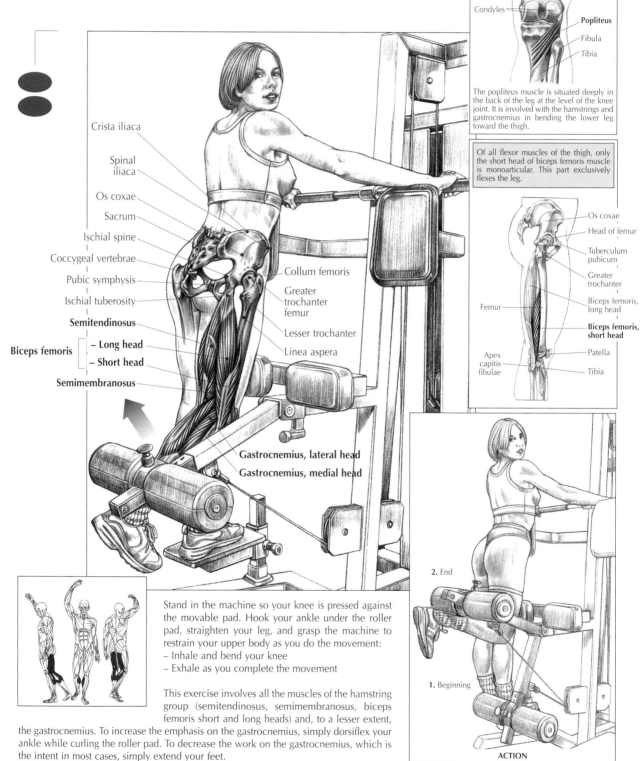

POPLITEUS MUSCLE

Femur
Condyles
Popliteus
Fibula
Tibia

The popliteus muscle is situated deeply in the back of the leg at the level of the knee joint. It is involved with the hamstrings and gastrocnemius in bending the lower leg toward the thigh.

Of all flexor muscles of the thigh, only the short head of biceps femoris muscle is monoarticular. This part exclusively flexes the leg.

Os coxae
Head of femur
Tuberculum pubicum
Greater trochanter
Biceps femoris, long head
Femur
Biceps femoris, short head
Apex capitis fibulae
Patella
Tibia

Crista iliaca
Spinal iliaca
Os coxae
Sacrum
Ischial spine
Coccygeal vertebrae
Pubic symphysis
Ischial tuberosity
Semitendinosus
Biceps femoris [**– Long head**
– Short head
Semimembranosus

Collum femoris
Greater trochanter femur
Lesser trochanter
Linea aspera

Gastrocnemius, lateral head
Gastrocnemius, medial head

2. End

1. Beginning

Stand in the machine so your knee is pressed against the movable pad. Hook your ankle under the roller pad, straighten your leg, and grasp the machine to restrain your upper body as you do the movement:
– Inhale and bend your knee
– Exhale as you complete the movement

This exercise involves all the muscles of the hamstring group (semitendinosus, semimembranosus, biceps femoris short and long heads) and, to a lesser extent, the gastrocnemius. To increase the emphasis on the gastrocnemius, simply dorsiflex your ankle while curling the roller pad. To decrease the work on the gastrocnemius, which is the intent in most cases, simply extend your feet.

ACTION

SEATED LEG CURLS

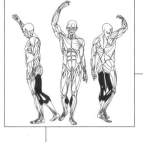

Peroneus tertius

Peroneus brevis

Soleus

Vastus intermedius

Tibialis anterior

Extensor digitorum longus

Patella

Peroneus longus

Quadriceps, rectus femoris

Obliquus externus abdominis

Tensior fasciae latae

Gluteus medius

Fascia lata, iliotibial tract

Greater trochanter

Gluteus maximus

Quadriceps femoris, vastus lateralis

Gastrocnemius — **Semimembranosus** — **Semitendinosus** — **Short head** — **Long head**

Biceps femoris

Biceps femoris, long head

Semitendinosus

Semi-membranosus

Biceps femoris, short head

Gastrocnemius, medial head

Gastrocnemius, lateral head

In the hamstring group, only the biceps femoris short head is monoarticular. It exclusively flexes the leg.

Sit on the machine with your legs straight, ankles resting on the roller pad. Lower the leg restraint over your thighs to secure them. Grasp the handles provided on each side:
– Inhale and bend your knees to move the roller pad downward
– Exhale as you complete the movement

This exercise works the hamstring group and, to a lesser extent, the gastrocnemius.

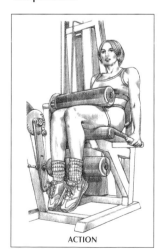

ACTION

11 GOOD MORNINGS

BEGINNING

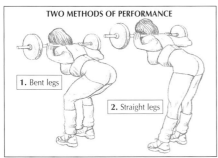

Keeping your legs straight while bending forward at the waist allows you to extend the hamstrings. You can better feel the hamstrings contracting as you straighten your upper body.

Keeping your knees flexed while bending forward at the waist allows you to relax the hamstrings, which makes hip flexion easier.

Latissimus dorsi

Musculi erectores spinale (under aponeurosis)

Obliquus externus abdominis

Gluteus medius

Gluteus maximus

Greater trochanter

Semitendinosus

Biceps femoris, long head

Semimembranosus

Biceps femoris, short head

Gastrocnemius, medial head

Gastrocnemius, lateral head

Soleus

Tensor fasciae latae

Quadriceps femoris, rectus femoris

Fascia lata

Quadriceps femoris, vastus lateralis

Patella

Tibialis anterior

Extensor digitorum longus

Peroneus longus

Peroneus brevis

TWO METHODS OF PERFORMANCE

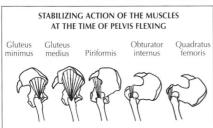

1. Bent legs

2. Straight legs

STABILIZING ACTION OF THE MUSCLES AT THE TIME OF PELVIS FLEXING

Gluteus minimus | Gluteus medius | Piriformis | Obturator internus | Quadratus femoris

Stand with your feet slightly apart. Place a barbell across your trapezius muscles or a little lower across your posterior deltoids:
– Inhale and bend forward at the waist until your torso is roughly parallel to the floor, being sure to keep your back straight
– Return to the starting position, exhaling

To make the movement easier, you can slightly bend your knees. This exercise involves the gluteals and spinal erectors, and particularly the hamstrings (except the biceps femoris short head, which only flexes the leg). Besides flexing the knee, the main function of the hamstrings is tilting the pelvis backward, straightening the upper body if the latest interact to contract the abdominals and sacrospinalis isometrically.

To get better construction in the hamstrings, never do this movement with heavy weight. In this exercise, the negative phase is excellent for stretching the back of your thighs. If you do it regularly, it will reduce the likelihood of injury when doing heavy squats.

This exercise does pose a high risk to the lumbar spine, so perform it with caution.

ACTION OF GLUTEUS MAXIMUS AND THE HAMSTRINGS DURING PELVIS STRAIGHTENING

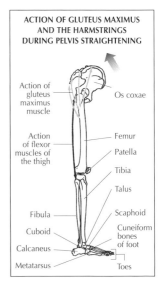

Action of gluteus maximus muscle

Action of flexor muscles of the thigh

Os coxae

Femur

Patella

Tibia

Talus

Fibula

Cuboid

Calcaneus

Metatarsus

Scaphoid

Cuneiform bones of foot

Toes

CABLE ADDUCTIONS 12

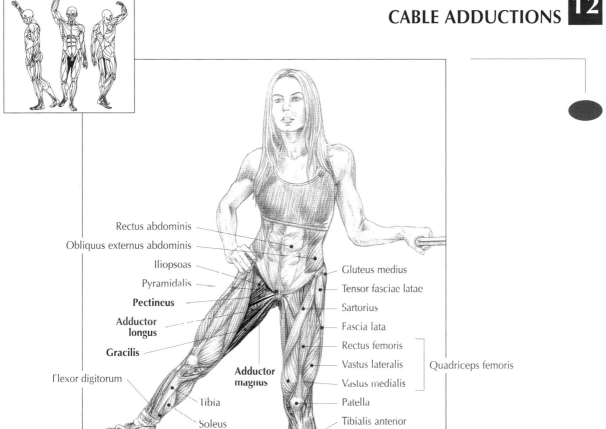

Rectus abdominis
Obliquus externus abdominis
Iliopsoas
Pyramidalis
Pectineus
Adductor longus
Gracilis
Flexor digitorum
Tibia
Soleus
Adductor magnus
Gastrocnemius, medial head

Gluteus medius
Tensor fasciae latae
Sartorius
Fascia lata
Rectus femoris
Vastus lateralis
Vastus medialis
Quadriceps femoris
Patella
Tibialis anterior
Extensor digitorum longus
Peroneus longus

Fasten the cuff to your ankle and grasp a fixed part of the machine with your opposite hand for support:
– Bring your leg attached to the cable toward and then across the other leg
– Return to the starting position

This exercise involves all the adductors (pectineus, adductor longus, adductor magnus and gracilis). It is an excellent movement for building the inner thighs.

13 MACHINE ADDUCTIONS

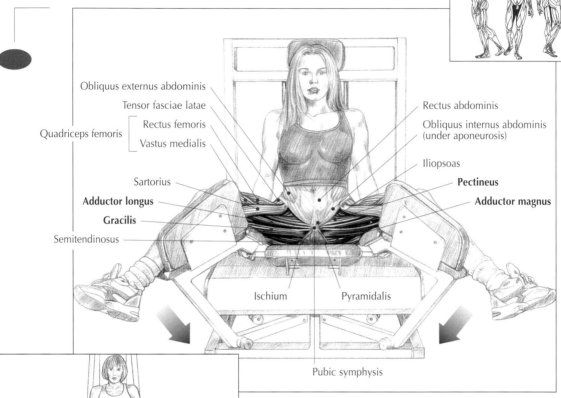

Obliquus externus abdominis
Tensor fasciae latae
Rectus femoris
Vastus medialis
Quadriceps femoris
Sartorius
Adductor longus
Gracilis
Semitendinosus

Rectus abdominis
Obliquus internus abdominis (under aponeurosis)
Iliopsoas
Pectineus
Adductor magnus

Ischium   Pyramidalis

Pubic symphysis

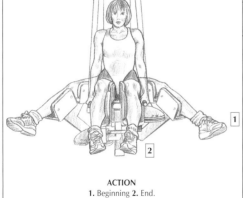

ACTION
1. Beginning **2.** End.

Sit on the machine with your legs spread:
– Force your thighs together
– Slowly return to the starting position

This exercise works the adductors (pectineus, adductor longus, adductor magnus, and gracilis). You can use heavier weight than with the cable adductions, but the range of movement will be more limited.

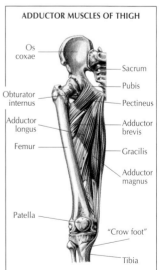

ADDUCTOR MUSCLES OF THIGH

Os coxae
Obturator internus
Adductor longus
Femur
Patella

Sacrum
Pubis
Pectineus
Adductor brevis
Gracilis
Adductor magnus
"Crow foot"
Tibia

STANDING CALF RAISES 14

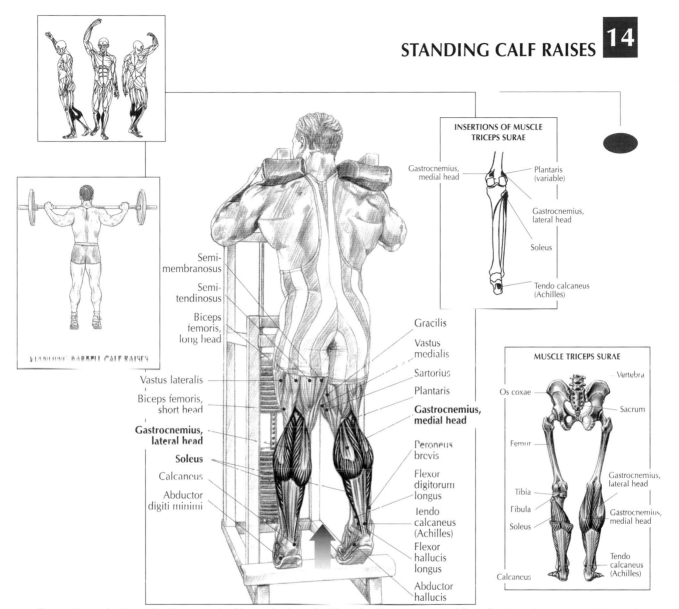

INSERTIONS OF MUSCLE TRICEPS SURAE

Gastrocnemius, medial head
Plantaris (variable)
Gastrocnemius, lateral head
Soleus
Tendo calcaneus (Achilles)

Semi-membranosus
Semi-tendinosus
Biceps femoris, long head
Vastus lateralis
Biceps femoris, short head
Gastrocnemius, lateral head
Soleus
Calcaneus
Abductor digiti minimi

Gracilis
Vastus medialis
Sartorius
Plantaris
Gastrocnemius, medial head
Peroneus brevis
Flexor digitorum longus
Tendo calcaneus (Achilles)
Flexor hallucis longus
Abductor hallucis

STANDING BARBELL CALF RAISES

MUSCLE TRICEPS SURAE

Vertebra
Os coxae
Sacrum
Femur
Gastrocnemius, lateral head
Tibia
Fibula
Soleus
Gastrocnemius, medial head
Calcaneus
Tendo calcaneus (Achilles)

Stand with your back straight. Place your shoulders under the pads of the yoke. Place your toes and the balls of your feet on the toe block and lower your heels (dorsiflexion):
– Rise up as high as you can on your toes (plantarflexion) while keeping your knees extended
– Return to the starting position

This exercise works the triceps surae (composed of the soleus and gastrocnemius, lateral and medial heads). To stretch your muscles correctly, be sure to rise up as high as possible on your toes as you perform every repetition. In theory, it is possible to isolate the stress on the gastrocnemius medial head (toes out) or on the gastrocnemius lateral head (toes in), but in practice, this is difficult to achieve. However, you can easily shift the emphasis from the gastrocnemius to the soleus by flexing your knees to relax the gastrocnemius.

Variation: you may also do this exercise at the Smith-machine, using a block or plates under your toes for greater range of motion. You may also place a bar on your shoulders, without the block, but thus, with a lesser range of motion.

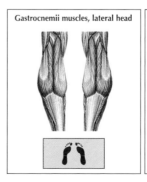

Gastrocnemii muscles, lateral head

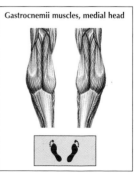

Gastrocnemii muscles, medial head

15 ONE-LEG TOE RAISES

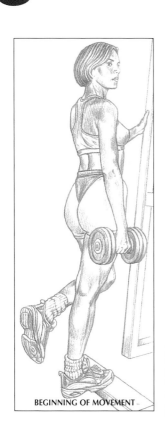

BEGINNING OF MOVEMENT

Biceps femoris, long head
Semitendinosus
Biceps femoris, short head
Semimembranosus

Triceps surae
– Gastrocnemius, lateral head
– Gastrocnemius, medial head
– Soleus

Tendo calcaneus
Calcaneus

Fascia lata
Vastus externalis
Crural
Patella
Peroneus longus
Extensor digitorum
Peroneus brevis
Extensor hallucis longus
Peroneus lateral malleolus

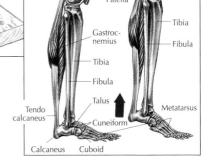

Femur
Femur
Patella
Tibia
Fibula
Gastroc-nemius
Tibia
Fibula
Tendo calcaneus
Talus
Metatarsus
Cuneiform
Calcaneus   Cuboid

Stand on one foot, placing the toes and ball of your foot on the toe block. Hold a dumbell in your hand on the same side as the foot you are standing on and grasp the edge of machine with your other hand to steady your body in position throughout the movement.
– Rise up as high as you can on your toes (plantarflexion), keeping your knee extented or very slightly bent
– Return to the starting position

This exercise works the triceps surae (composed of the soleus and gastrocnemius lateral and medial heads). Make sure you flex your foot completely as you perform every repetition in order to stretch the triceps surae correctly. For the best results, do only long sets until you feel the burning sensation.

DONKEY CALF RAISES 16

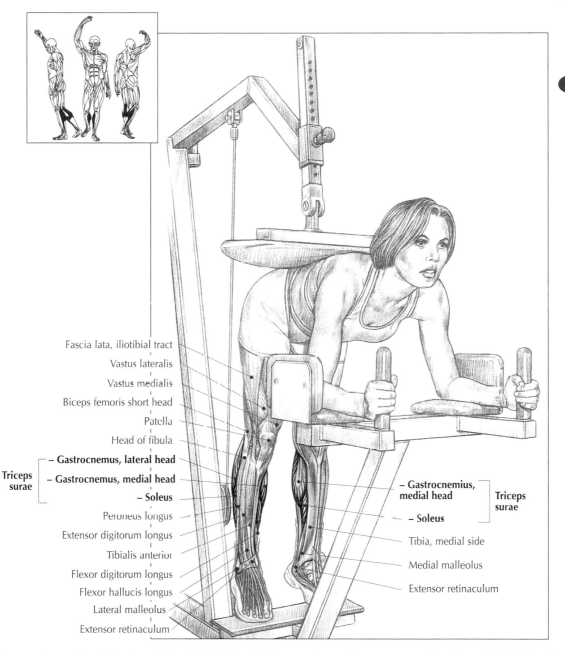

Fascia lata, iliotibial tract
Vastus lateralis
Vastus medialis
Biceps femoris short head
Patella
Head of fibula
Triceps surae { **– Gastrocnemius, lateral head**
– Gastrocnemius, medial head
– Soleus
Peroneus longus
Extensor digitorum longus
Tibialis anterior
Flexor digitorum longus
Flexor hallucis longus
Lateral malleolus
Extensor retinaculum

– Gastrocnemius, medial head
– Soleus } **Triceps surae**
Tibia, medial side
Medial malleolus
Extensor retinaculum

Place your toes and the balls of your feet on the footplate, straighten your legs, and lean over so your torso is parallel to the floor. Rest your forearms on the front support and press your pelvis against the padded surface of the machine:
– Drop your heels as far below your toes as possible (dorsiflexion)
– Rise up as high as you can on your toes until your calves are fully flexed (plantarflexion)

This exercise works the triceps surae. With the knee flexed, it emphasizes the soleus.

Variation: you can also arrange a toe block close enough to a flat exercise bench so you can place your toes on the block, lean over having your torso parallel to the floor, and rest your forearms on the bench. For resistance, have a training partner climb up astride your hips as if riding a horse.

17 SEATED CALF RAISES

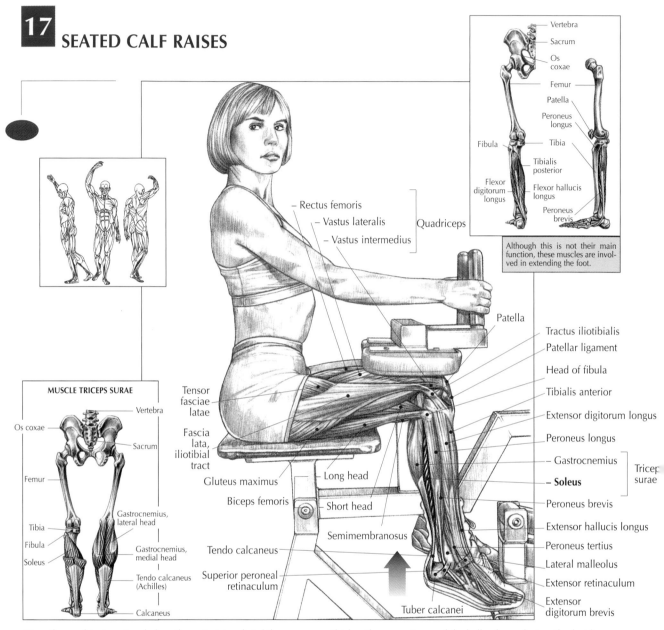

Vertebra
Sacrum
Os coxae
Femur
Patella
Peroneus longus
Fibula
Tibia
Tibialis posterior
Flexor digitorum longus
Flexor hallucis longus
Peroneus brevis

Although this is not their main function, these muscles are involved in extending the foot.

– Rectus femoris
– Vastus lateralis
– Vastus intermedius
Quadriceps

Patella
Tractus iliotibialis
Patellar ligament
Head of fibula
Tibialis anterior
Extensor digitorum longus
Peroneus longus
– Gastrocnemius
– **Soleus**
Triceps surae
Peroneus brevis
Extensor hallucis longus
Peroneus tertius
Lateral malleolus
Extensor retinaculum
Extensor digitorum brevis

Tensor fasciae latae
Fascia lata, iliotibial tract
Gluteus maximus
Biceps femoris
Long head
Short head
Semimembranosus
Tendo calcaneus
Superior peroneal retinaculum
Tuber calcanei

MUSCLE TRICEPS SURAE

Vertebra
Os coxae
Sacrum
Femur
Gastrocnemius, lateral head
Tibia
Fibula
Soleus
Gastrocnemius, medial head
Tendo calcaneus (Achilles)
Calcaneus

Sit on the machine's seat and place the restraint pads tightly across your thighs. Place your toes and the balls of your feet on the foot bar:
– Stretch your heels as far below the level of your toes as possible (dorsiflexion)
– Rise up as high as you can under resistance on your toes (plantarflexion)

This exercise places primary emphasis on the soleus (muscle lying immediately below the gastrocnemius, attached under the knee joint and connected with the calcaneus via the Achilles tendon; the function of the soleus and gastrocnemius is to extend the ankle).
Bending your legs relaxes the gastrocnemius. Therefore, the gastrocnemius is only slightly stressed when you extend your foot.

Variation: sit on a bench with your toes and the balls of your feet on a toe block. Pad the middle of a barbell handle (by rolling a towel around it) and rest the barbell across your knees to simulate this movement.

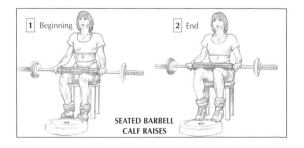

1 Beginning   2 End

SEATED BARBELL CALF RAISES

SEATED BARBELL CALF RAISES 18

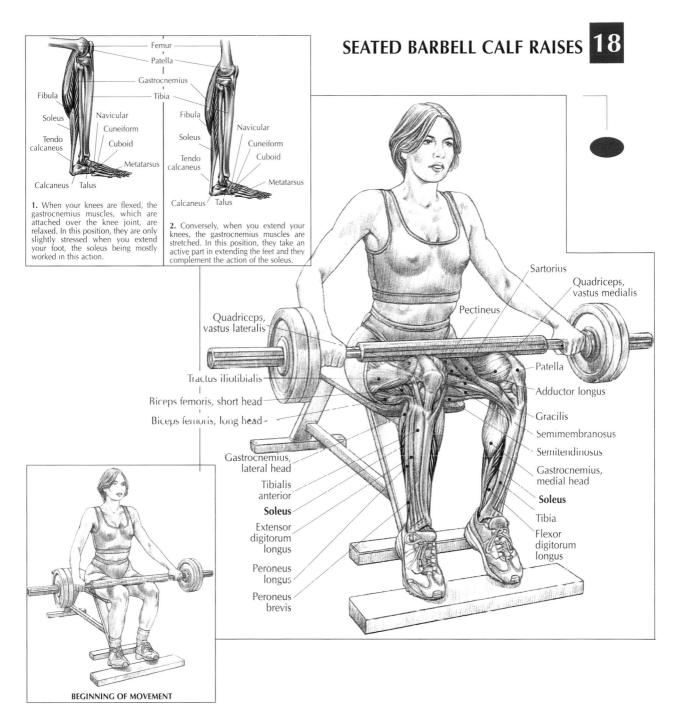

Femur
Patella
Gastrocnemius
Fibula
Tibia
Soleus
Navicular
Cuneiform
Tendo calcaneus
Cuboid
Metatarsus
Calcaneus
Talus

1. When your knees are flexed, the gastrocnemius muscles, which are attached over the knee joint, are relaxed. In this position, they are only slightly stressed when you extend your foot, the soleus being mostly worked in this action.

Fibula
Navicular
Soleus
Cuneiform
Cuboid
Tendo calcaneus
Metatarsus
Calcaneus
Talus

2. Conversely, when you extend your knees, the gastrocnemius muscles are stretched. In this position, they take an active part in extending the feet and they complement the action of the soleus.

Sartorius
Quadriceps, vastus medialis
Pectineus
Quadriceps, vastus lateralis
Patella
Adductor longus
Tractus iliotibialis
Gracilis
Biceps femoris, short head
Semimembranosus
Biceps femoris, long head
Semitendinosus
Gastrocnemius, medial head
Gastrocnemius, lateral head
Soleus
Tibialis anterior
Tibia
Soleus
Flexor digitorum longus
Extensor digitorum longus
Peroneus longus
Peroneus brevis

BEGINNING OF MOVEMENT

Sit on a bench. Place your toes and the balls of your feet on a toe block:
– Rest the barbell across your lower thighs
– Push down with your toes and extend your feet as completely as possible (plantarflexion)

This exercise isolates the soleus, which belongs to the triceps surae. It is attached under the knee joint on the shin and fibula and it is connected to the calcaneus (via the Achilles tendon). Its function is to extend the ankles. Unlike seated machine calf raises, which allow you to work with heavy weight, you won't be able to do this movement with heavy weight because it will be difficult to load.

Variation: you can do this movement on a chair or a bench without adding weight. In that case, do long sets until you feel the burning sensation.

6 BUTTOCKS

1. Lunges
2. Cable Kick Backs
3. Machine Hip Extensions (Kick Backs)
4. Floor Hip Extensions(Kick Backs)
5. Bridging
6. Cable Hip Abductions
7. Standing Machine Hip Abductions
8. Floor Hip Abductions
9. Seated Machine Hip Abductions

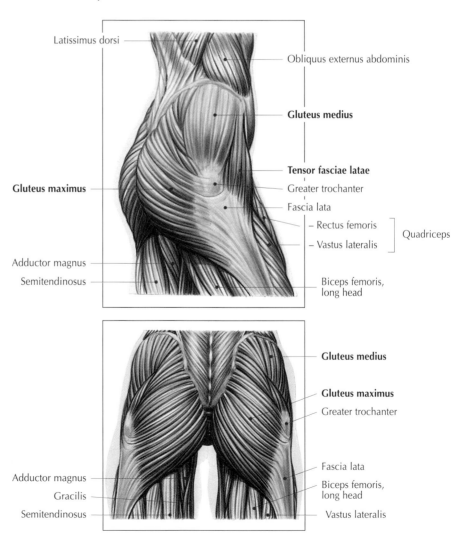

LUNGES 1

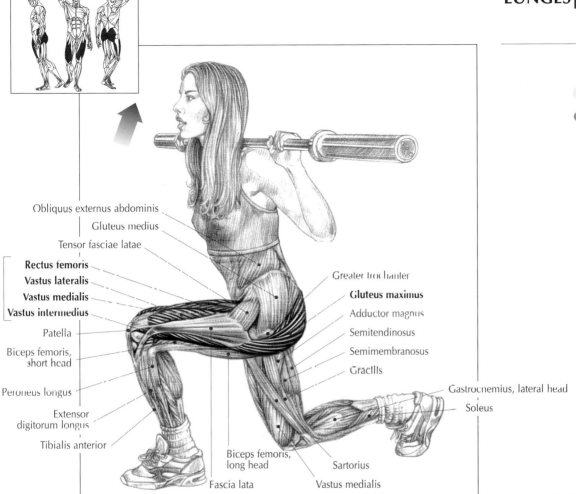

Obliquus externus abdominis
Gluteus medius
Tensor fasciae latae
Rectus femoris
Vastus lateralis
Vastus medialis
Vastus intermedius
Patella
Biceps femoris, short head
Peroneus longus
Extensor digitorum longus
Tibialis anterior

driceps

Greater trochanter
Gluteus maximus
Adductor magnus
Semitendinosus
Semimembranosus
Gracilis
Gastrocnemius, lateral head
Soleus

Biceps femoris, long head
Fascia lata
Sartorius
Vastus medialis

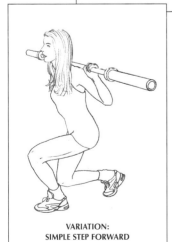

**VARIATION:
SIMPLE STEP FORWARD**

Stand with your feet hip-width apart. Lift a light barbell up to a position across your shoulders behind your neck:
– Inhale and take a comfortable step forward, keeping your torso as upright as possible
– In the bottom position, the top of your forward thigh is slightly below parallel
– Return to the starting position, exhaling

This exercise places primary emphasis on the gluteals. You can vary the stride length by taking (1) a simple step forward to specifically involve the quadriceps, or (2) a large step forward to place more stress on the hamstrings and gluteals while stretching the upper quadriceps and hip flexors of the back leg.

Note: as you lunge forward, you put all of your body weight on your leading leg. It is a relatively difficult exercise to perform because of the balance required. Beginners should start with very light weight.

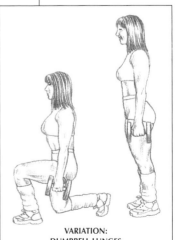

**VARIATION:
DUMBBELL LUNGES**

2 CABLE BACK KICKS

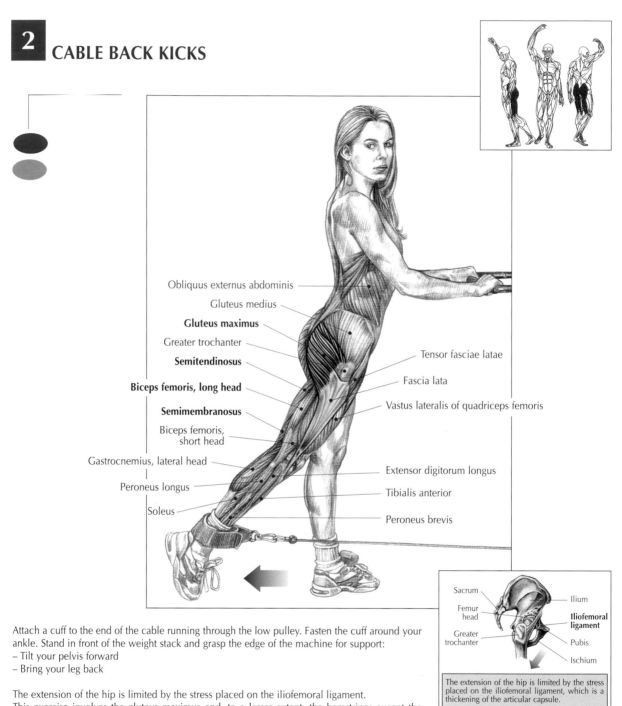

Obliquus externus abdominis

Gluteus medius

Gluteus maximus

Greater trochanter

Semitendinosus

Biceps femoris, long head

Semimembranosus

Biceps femoris, short head

Gastrocnemius, lateral head

Peroneus longus

Soleus

Tensor fasciae latae

Fascia lata

Vastus lateralis of quadriceps femoris

Extensor digitorum longus

Tibialis anterior

Peroneus brevis

Sacrum

Femur head

Greater trochanter

Ilium

Iliofemoral ligament

Pubis

Ischium

The extension of the hip is limited by the stress placed on the iliofemoral ligament, which is a thickening of the articular capsule.

Attach a cuff to the end of the cable running through the low pulley. Fasten the cuff around your ankle. Stand in front of the weight stack and grasp the edge of the machine for support:
– Tilt your pelvis forward
– Bring your leg back

The extension of the hip is limited by the stress placed on the iliofemoral ligament.
This exercise involves the gluteus maximus and, to a lesser extent, the hamstrings except the biceps femoris short head. This exercise allows you to develop shapely legs while increasing muscle tone to your gluteals.

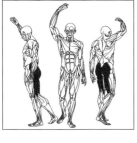

MACHINE HIP EXTENSIONS 3

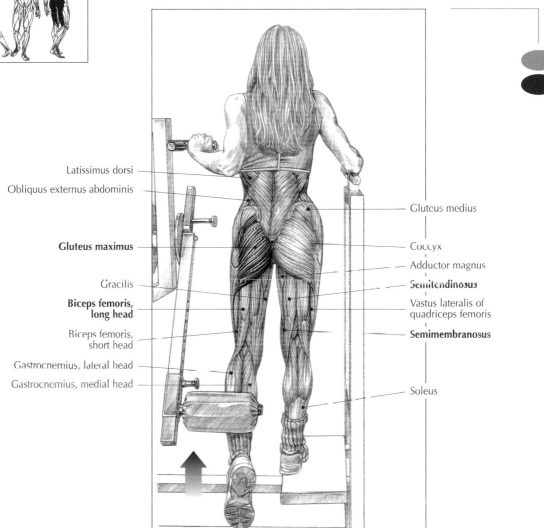

Latissimus dorsi
Obliquus externus abdominis

Gluteus maximus

Gracilis

Biceps femoris, long head

Biceps femoris, short head

Gastrocnemius, lateral head
Gastrocnemius, medial head

Gluteus medius

Coccyx
Adductor magnus
Semitendinosus
Vastus lateralis of quadriceps femoris
Semimembranosus

Soleus

Grasp the handles of the machine, place one foot on the footplate and bring your opposite leg slightly forward, with the pad halfway between knee joint and ankle. Bend forward slightly:
– Inhale and move your thigh to the rear until your hip is fully extended backward (hyperextension)
– Hold this peak contracted position for 2 seconds and return to the starting position
– Exhale as you complete the extension

This exercise works the gluteals, and, to a lesser extent, the semitendinosus, semimembranosus, and biceps femoris long head.

4 FLOOR HIP EXTENSIONS

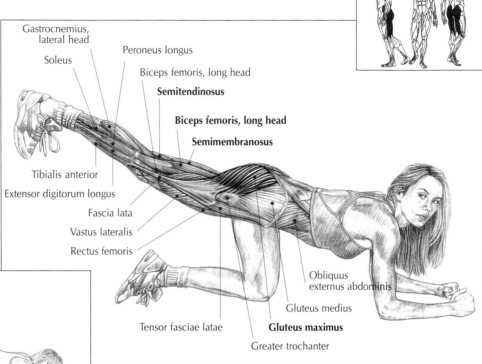

Gastrocnemius, lateral head
Soleus
Peroneus longus
Biceps femoris, long head
Semitendinosus
Biceps femoris, long head
Semimembranosus
Tibialis anterior
Extensor digitorum longus
Fascia lata
Vastus lateralis
Rectus femoris
Obliquus externus abdominis
Gluteus medius
Tensor fasciae latae
Gluteus maximus
Greater trochanter

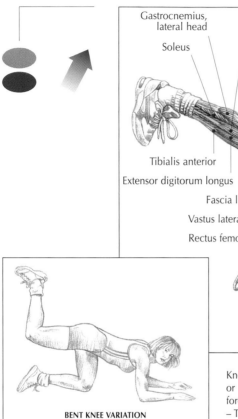

BENT KNEE VARIATION

Kneel on one leg with your elbows or hands on the floor and your forearms straight:
– Tuck your opposite leg under your chest
– Move your tucked leg to the rear until your hip is fully extended

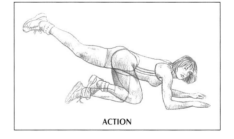

ACTION

If you swing your leg to a straightened position, the exercise will work the hamstrings and gluteals ; if you keep your knee bent, it will only work the gluteals, but less intensely.
You can increase the range of motion or limit it at the end of the extension. You can hold a peak contracted position for a couple of seconds at the end of the movement. For more intensity, strap a soft weight around your ankle. This exercise is very easy to perform and gives good results. It has become very popular and is often used in aerobics classes.

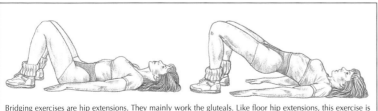

Bridging exercises are hip extensions. They mainly work the gluteals. Like floor hip extensions, this exercise is done without weight and can be performed anywhere.

BRIDGING 5

– Rectus femoris
– Vastus lateralis
– Vastus medialis
– Vastus intermedius
Quadriceps femoris

Fascia lata
Greater trochanter
Tensor fasciae latae
Gluteus maximus
Gluteus medius
Crista iliaca
Obliquus externus abdominis

Patella
– Short head
– Long head
Biceps femoris
Peroneus longus
Soleus
Peroneus brevis
Gastrocnemius, lateral head

Lie on the floor with your entire spine in contact with the floor. Place your hands on the floor next to your hips. Flex your knees to 90 degrees:
– ILift your buttocks off the floor, pushing with your feet as high as you can
– Hold the position for 2 seconds and lower your pelvis without putting your buttocks back on the floor
– Immediately repeat

This exercise works the hamstrings and gluteals.
Make sure you correctly feel the muscle contraction at the end of every repetition.

Note: this easy exercise has proved beneficial. It is performed in most aerobics classes.

BEGINNING OF MOVEMENT

VARIATION ON THE BENCH

BEGINNING OF MOVEMENT

Variations:
1. You can do the movement with a limited range of motion.
2. For more intensity, you can put your feet on a bench.

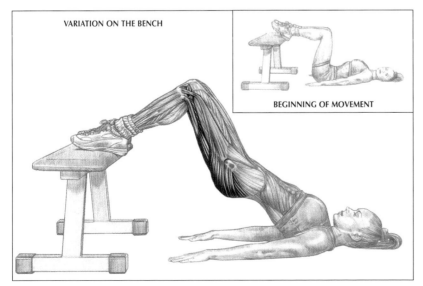

6 CABLE HIP ABDUCTIONS

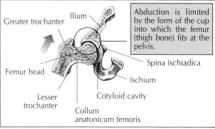

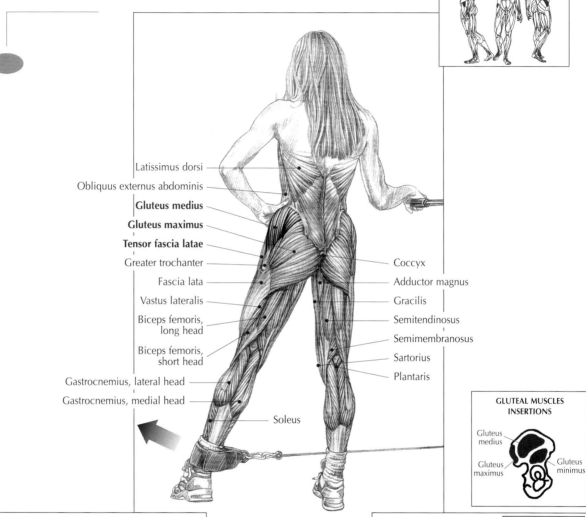

Latissimus dorsi

Obliquus externus abdominis

Gluteus medius

Gluteus maximus

Tensor fascia latae

Greater trochanter

Fascia lata

Vastus lateralis

Biceps femoris, long head

Biceps femoris, short head

Gastrocnemius, lateral head

Gastrocnemius, medial head

Soleus

Coccyx

Adductor magnus

Gracilis

Semitendinosus

Semimembranosus

Sartorius

Plantaris

GLUTEAL MUSCLES INSERTIONS

Gluteus medius

Gluteus maximus

Gluteus minimus

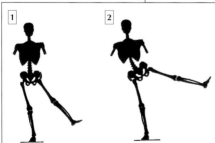

1. Hip abduction (limited by the shape of the pelvic cup into which the thigh bone fits).
2. Forced hip abduction (tilt of the pelvis to the opposite femoral head).

Attach a low pulley to your ankle:
– Grasp the edge of the machine with your opposite hand to stabilize your body.
– Raise laterly your leg as far as you can.

This exercise involves the gluteus maximus, the deeper gluteus minimus, and tensor fascia latae.

Greater trochanter

Ilium

Femur head

Lesser trochanter

Collum anatonicum femoris

Spina ischiadica

Ischium

Cotyloid cavity

Abduction is limited by the form of the cup into which the femur (thigh bone) fits at the pelvis.

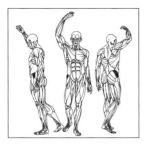

STANDING MACHINE HIP ABDUCTIONS 7

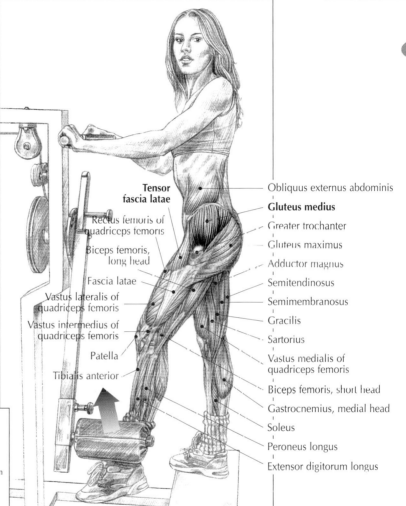

Tensor
fascia latae — Obliquus externus abdominis

Rectus femoris of — **Gluteus medius**
quadriceps femoris Greater trochanter

Biceps femoris, Gluteus maximus
long head Adductor magnus

Fascia latae Semitendinosus

Vastus lateralis of Semimembranosus
quadriceps femoris
Gracilis
Vastus intermedius of
quadriceps femoris Sartorius

Patella Vastus medialis of
quadriceps femoris
Tibialis anterior
Biceps femoris, short head

Gastrocnemius, medial head

Soleus

Peroneus longus

Extensor digitorum longus

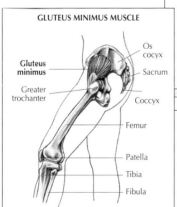

GLUTEUS MINIMUS MUSCLE

Os
cocyx
**Gluteus
minimus** Sacrum

Greater
trochanter Coccyx

Femur

Patella

Tibia

Fibula

Place one foot on the footplate and place the outer side of your other leg against the pad below your knee (close to your ankle):
– Move this leg as high to the side as possible
– Note the abduction is limited because the neck of the femur (thigh bone) is rapidly stopped on the rim of the cup into which the femur fits at the pelvis

This exercise is excellent for developing the gluteus medius and the gluteus minimus, which has the same function as the anterior fibers of the gluteus medius. It also works tensor fascia latae.

8 FLOOR HIP ABDUCTIONS

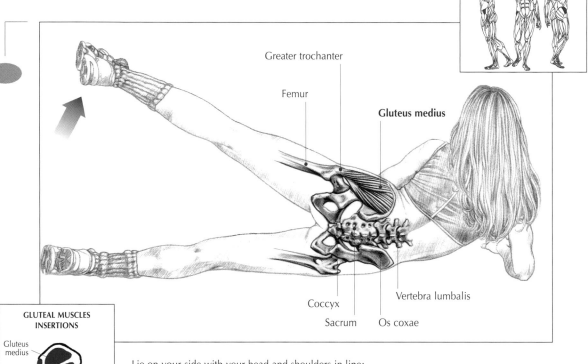

Greater trochanter

Femur

Gluteus medius

Vertebra lumbalis

Coccyx

Sacrum

Os coxae

GLUTEAL MUSCLES INSERTIONS

Gluteus medius

Gluteus minimum

Gluteus maxiumus

Lie on your side with your head and shoulders in line:
– Lift your leg to an angle of 70 degrees (at the most) off the floor, always keeping your knee extended
– Return to the starting position and repeat

This exercise involves the gluteus medius and gluteus minimus. You can increase or decrease the range of motion. Hold a peak contracted position for a couple seconds at the end of the abduction. You can raise your leg lither slightly forward, slightly backward, or vertically. For more resistance, strap a soft weight around your ankle or use a low pulley.

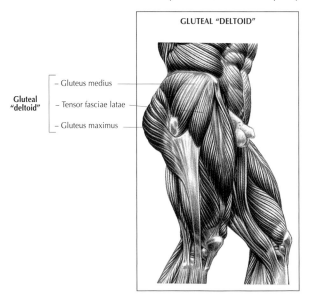

GLUTEAL "DELTOID"

Gluteal "deltoid"

– Gluteus medius
– Tensor fasciae latae
– Gluteus maximus

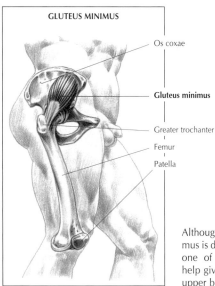

GLUTEUS MINIMUS

Os coxae

Gluteus minimus

Greater trochanter

Femur

Patella

Although the gluteus minimus is deeply situated, it is one of the muscles that help give more size to the upper buttocks.

SEATED MACHINE HIP ABDUCTIONS 9

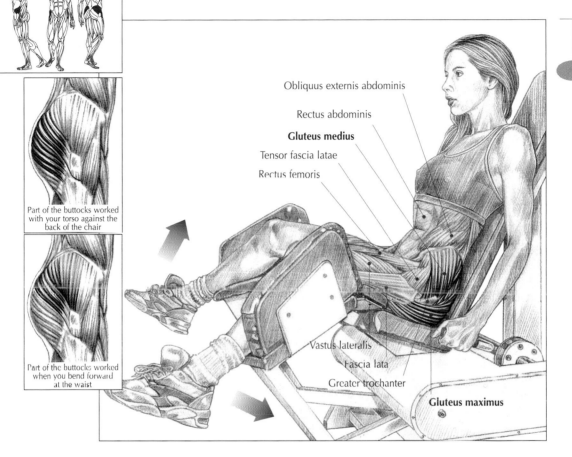

Obliquus externis abdominis

Rectus abdominis

Gluteus medius

Tensor fascia latae

Rectus femoris

Vastus lateralis

Fascia lata

Greater trochanter

Gluteus maximus

Part of the buttocks worked with your torso against the back of the chair

Part of the buttocks worked when you bend forward at the waist

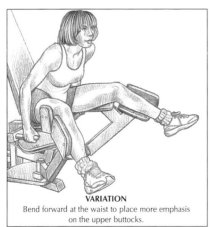

VARIATION
Bend forward at the waist to place more emphasis on the upper buttocks.

Sit at an abductor machine:
– Slowly force your legs apart as far as comfortably possible
– Return to the starting position and repeat

If the machine's seat is inclined, you will work the gluteus medius. If the machine's seat is upright, you will work the gluteus maximus. Ideally, you should vary the inclination of your torso in every set. Simply bend at the waist. For example: 10 reps with upper body against the back of the seat followed by 10 reps with upper body bent forward at the waist.

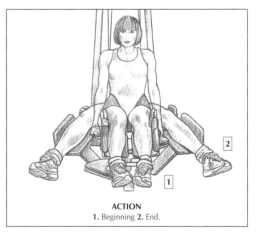

ACTION
1. Beginning 2. End.

This exercise is an excellent way to increase muscle tone to the upper part of the hip. It gives the buttocks a rounded appearance, making your waist look slimmer.

7 ABDOMEN

1. Crunches
2. Sit-Ups
3. Gym Ladder Sit-Ups
4. Calves Over Bench Sit-Ups
5. Incline Bench Sit-Ups
6. Specific Bench Sit-Ups
7. High Pulley Crunches
8. Machine Crunches
9. Incline Leg Raises
10. Leg Raises
11. Hanging Leg Raises
12. Broomstick Twists
13. Dumbbell Side Bends
14. Roman Chair Side Bends
15. Machine Trunk Rotations

Although this is a much-debated topic, if you have lower back problems, you should keep your hip motionless in order to neutralize the action of the psoas and prevent abnormal forward curvature of the spine (lordosis) or other spinal pathologies. Therefore, it is better to stress the rectus abdominis without stretching them, by moving the sternum (breastbone) closer to the pubis with short contractions.

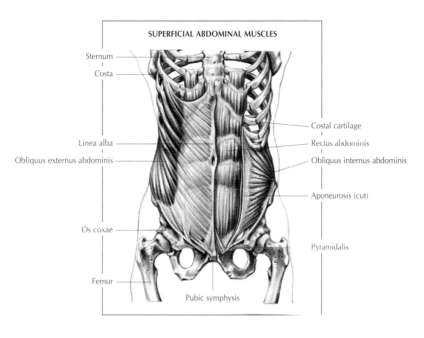

SUPERFICIAL ABDOMINAL MUSCLES

Sternum
Costa
Linea alba
Obliquus externus abdominis
Os coxae
Femur
Pubic symphysis
Costal cartilage
Rectus abdominis
Obliquus internus abdominis
Aponeurosis (cut)
Pyramidalis

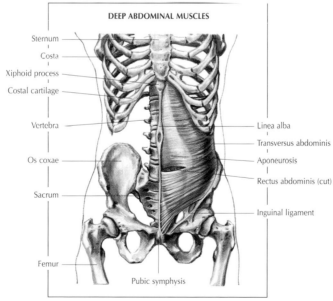

DEEP ABDOMINAL MUSCLES

Sternum
Costa
Xiphoid process
Costal cartilage
Vertebra
Os coxae
Sacrum
Femur
Pubic symphysis
Linea alba
Transversus abdominis
Aponeurosis
Rectus abdominis (cut)
Inguinal ligament

1 CRUNCHES

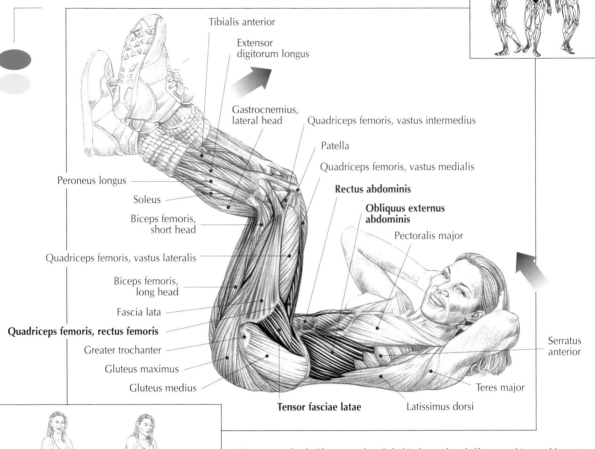

Tibialis anterior
Extensor digitorum longus
Gastrocnemius, lateral head
Quadriceps femoris, vastus intermedius
Patella
Quadriceps femoris, vastus medialis
Rectus abdominis
Obliquus externus abdominis
Pectoralis major

Peroneus longus
Soleus
Biceps femoris, short head
Quadriceps femoris, vastus lateralis
Biceps femoris, long head
Fascia lata
Quadriceps femoris, rectus femoris
Greater trochanter
Gluteus maximus
Gluteus medius

Tensor fasciae latae
Latissimus dorsi
Teres major
Serratus anterior

VARIATION : seated flat bench crunches.

Lie on your back. Place your hands behind your head. Flex your hips and knees to a 90 degrees angle:
– Inhale and lift your shoulders off the floor, moving your knees closer to your head by shortening your torso
– Exhale as you complete the movement

This exercise particularly works the rectus abdominis. To place more emphasis on the obliques, simply twist alternately from side to side (move your right elbow to your left knee, then move your left elbow to your right knee, and so on).

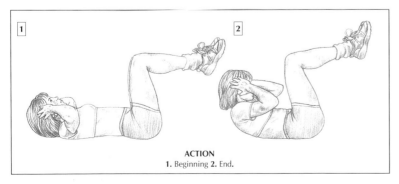

1   2

ACTION
1. Beginning **2.** End.

The object of the crunch is to shorten your torso, moving your pubis closer to your breastbone by deliberately contracting your abdominals.

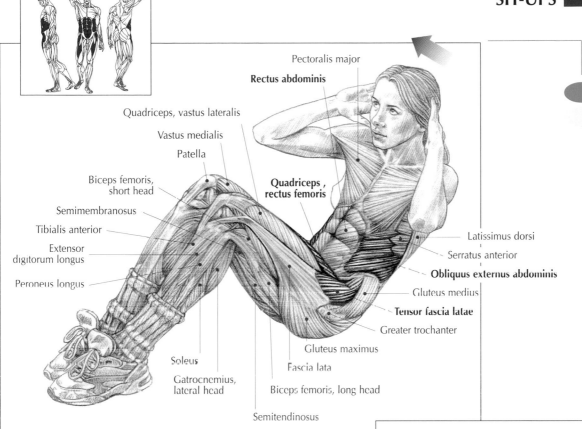

Pectoralis major

Rectus abdominis

Quadriceps, vastus lateralis

Vastus medialis

Patella

Biceps femoris, short head

Semimembranosus

Tibialis anterior

Extensor digitorum longus

Peroneus longus

Quadriceps, rectus femoris

Latissimus dorsi

Serratus anterior

Obliquus externus abdominis

Gluteus medius

Tensor fascia latae

Greater trochanter

Gluteus maximus

Soleus

Gatrocnemius, lateral head

Biceps femoris, long head

Fascia lata

Semitendinosus

Lie on your back with your legs bent and your feet on the floor. Place your hands behind your head:
– Inhale and curl your torso off the floor
– Exhale as you complete the movement
– Return to the starting position without resting your torso on the floor
– Repeat until you feel the burning sensation coming from your abdominals

This exercise works the hip flexors, obliques, and focuses on the rectus abdominis.

Variations:
1. For more balance, ask a training partner to hold your feet.
2. To make it easier, extend your arms forward. This variation is recommended for beginners.

INCLINED BOARD VARIATION
To add resistance to your sit-ups, you can raise the board.

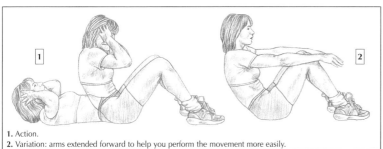

1. Action.
2. Variation: arms extended forward to help you perform the movement more easily.

3 GYM LADDER SIT-UPS

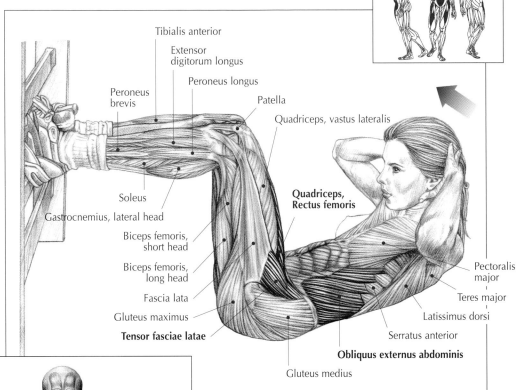

Tibialis anterior

Extensor
digitorum longus

Peroneus longus

Peroneus
brevis

Patella

Quadriceps, vastus lateralis

Soleus

**Quadriceps,
Rectus femoris**

Gastrocnemius, lateral head

Biceps femoris,
short head

Biceps femoris,
long head

Fascia lata

Gluteus maximus

Tensor fasciae latae

Gluteus medius

Pectoralis
major

Teres major

Latissimus dorsi

Serratus anterior

Obliquus externus abdominis

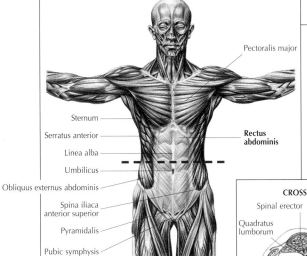

Pectoralis major

Sternum

Serratus anterior

Linea alba

Umbilicus

Obliquus externus abdominis

Spina iliaca
anterior superior

Pyramidalis

Pubic symphysis

**Rectus
abdominis**

Hook your feet in the gym ladder with your hips and knees flexed to 90 degrees. Place your hands behind your head:
– Inhale and curl your torso as high as possible off the floor
– Exhale as you complete the movement

This exercise focuses on the rectus abdominis and places secondary emphasis on the internal and external obliques.
Place your torso farther from the gym ladder and hook your feet lower to increase pelvic mobility, allowing a greater range of motion and more involvement of the hip flexors.

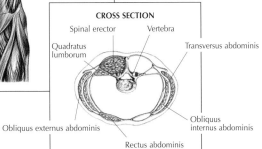

CROSS SECTION

Spinal erector

Vertebra

Quadratus
lumborum

Transversus abdominis

Obliquus externus abdominis

Obliquus
internus abdominis

Rectus abdominis

CALVES OVER BENCH SIT-UPS **4**

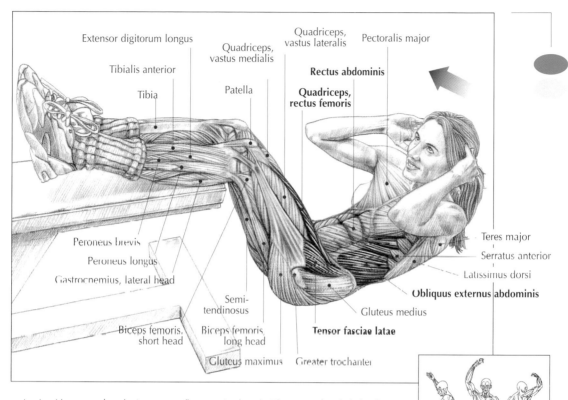

Extensor digitorum longus

Quadriceps,
vastus medialis

Quadriceps,
vastus lateralis

Pectoralis major

Tibialis anterior

Rectus abdominis

Tibia

Patella

**Quadriceps,
rectus femoris**

Teres major

Serratus anterior

Latissimus dorsi

Peroneus brevis

Peroneus longus

Gastrocnemius, lateral head

Semi-
tendinosus

Obliquus externus abdominis

Gluteus medius

Tensor fasciae latae

Biceps femoris,
short head

Biceps femoris,
long head

Gluteus maximus

Greater trochanter

Lie on your back with your calves laying over a flat exercise bench. Place your hands behind your head:
– Inhale and lift your shoulders off the floor
– Try to touch your knees with your head
– Exhale as you complete the movement

This exercise focuses on the rectus abdominis, particularly above the navel. By placing your torso farther from the bench you increase pelvic mobility which allows your torso upward by contracting the iliopsoas, tensor fasciae latae, and rectus femoris in order to flex the hips.

5 INCLINE BENCH SIT-UPS

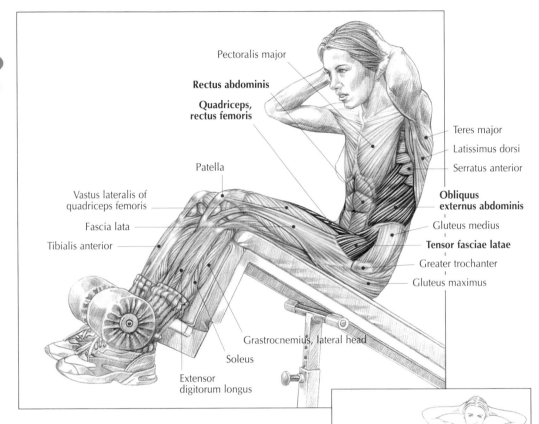

Pectoralis major

Rectus abdominis

Quadriceps, rectus femoris

Patella

Vastus lateralis of quadriceps femoris

Fascia lata

Tibialis anterior

Grastrocnemius, lateral head

Soleus

Extensor digitorum longus

Teres major

Latissimus dorsi

Serratus anterior

Obliquus externus abdominis

Gluteus medius

Tensor fasciae latae

Greater trochanter

Gluteus maximus

VARIATION WITH TRUNK ROTATION

Sit on the bench and hook your feet under the roller pads. Place your hands behind your neck:
– Inhale and incline your torso less than 20 degrees
– Move your torso back up, slightly curling your torso to place more stress on the rectus abdominis
– Exhale as you complete the movement

This exercise works the entire rectus abdominis muscle wall, as well as the iliop-soas, tensor fasciae latae, and rectus femoris in the quadriceps group. The func-tion of these last three muscles is to tilt the pelvis forward.

Variation: as you move back up, you can twist alternately to each side on suc-cessive repetitions to shift part of the stress to the obliques.

Example: twisting your torso to the left will more intensely involve the right external oblique, left internal oblique, and the right rectus abdo-minis.

This movement can be done twisting alternately or unilaterally for the required number of repetitions. In either case, you should concentrate on the movement as you do it until you feel the tension in your muscles. There is no advantage to excessively increasing the bench's incline.

SPECIFIC BENCH SIT-UPS **6**

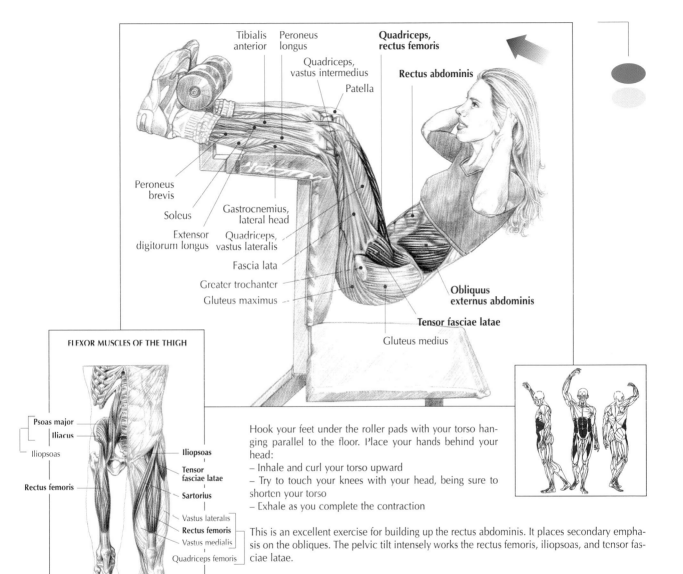

Tibialis anterior
Peroneus longus
Quadriceps, rectus femoris
Quadriceps, vastus intermedius
Rectus abdominis
Patella
Peroneus brevis
Soleus
Gastrocnemius, lateral head
Extensor digitorum longus
Quadriceps, vastus lateralis
Fascia lata
Greater trochanter
Gluteus maximus
Obliquus externus abdominis
Tensor fasciae latae
Gluteus medius

FLEXOR MUSCLES OF THE THIGH

Psoas major
Iliacus
Iliopsoas
Rectus femoris
Iliopsoas
Tensor fasciae latae
Sartorius
Vastus lateralis
Rectus femoris
Vastus medialis
Quadriceps femoris

Hook your feet under the roller pads with your torso hanging parallel to the floor. Place your hands behind your head:
– Inhale and curl your torso upward
– Try to touch your knees with your head, being sure to shorten your torso
– Exhale as you complete the contraction

This is an excellent exercise for building up the rectus abdominis. It places secondary emphasis on the obliques. The pelvic tilt intensely works the rectus femoris, iliopsoas, and tensor fasciae latae.

Note: beginners should start with easier exercises to gain the strength level required.

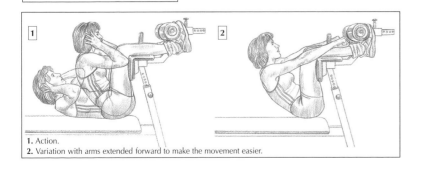

1. Action.
2. Variation with arms extended forward to make the movement easier.

7 HIGH PULLEY CRUNCHES

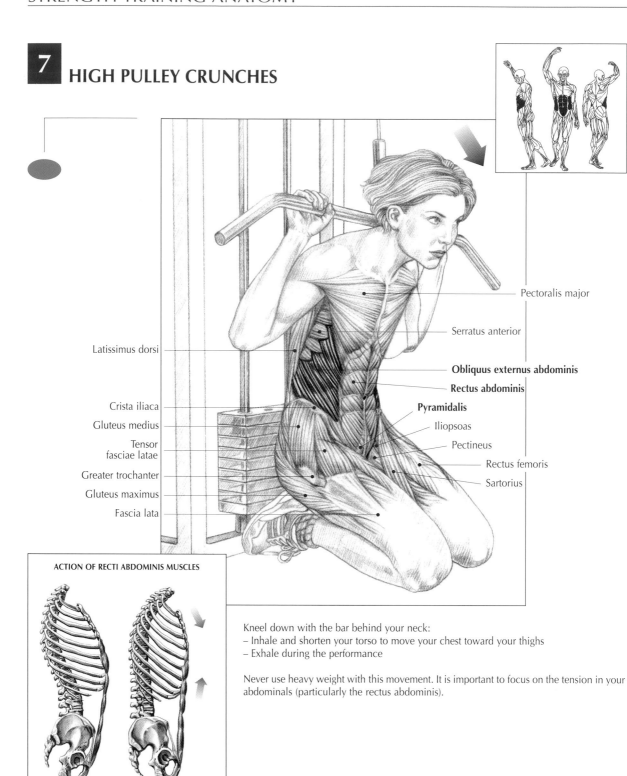

Pectoralis major

Serratus anterior

Obliquus externus abdominis

Rectus abdominis

Pyramidalis

Iliopsoas

Pectineus

Rectus femoris

Sartorius

Latissimus dorsi

Crista iliaca

Gluteus medius

Tensor fasciae latae

Greater trochanter

Gluteus maximus

Fascia lata

ACTION OF RECTI ABDOMINIS MUSCLES

Kneel down with the bar behind your neck:
– Inhale and shorten your torso to move your chest toward your thighs
– Exhale during the performance

Never use heavy weight with this movement. It is important to focus on the tension in your abdominals (particularly the rectus abdominis).

MACHINE CRUNCHES 8

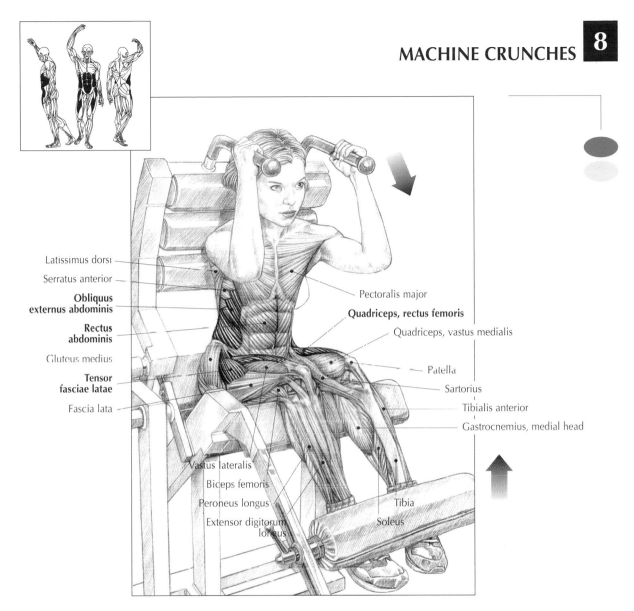

Latissimus dorsi

Serratus anterior

Obliquus externus abdominis

Rectus abdominis

Gluteus medius

Tensor fasciae latae

Fascia lata

Vastus lateralis

Biceps femoris

Peroneus longus

Extensor digitorum longus

Pectoralis major

Quadriceps, rectus femoris

Quadriceps, vastus medialis

Patella

Sartorius

Tibialis anterior

Gastrocnemius, medial head

Tibia

Soleus

Sit on the machine, grasp the handles, and hook your feet under the roller pad:
– Inhale and shorten your torso, trying to move your chest toward your thighs
– Exhale at the end of the movement

This excellent exercise allows you to select the weight. Beginners should start with light weight. Experienced athletes can safely work with heavy weight.

9 INCLINE LEG RAISES

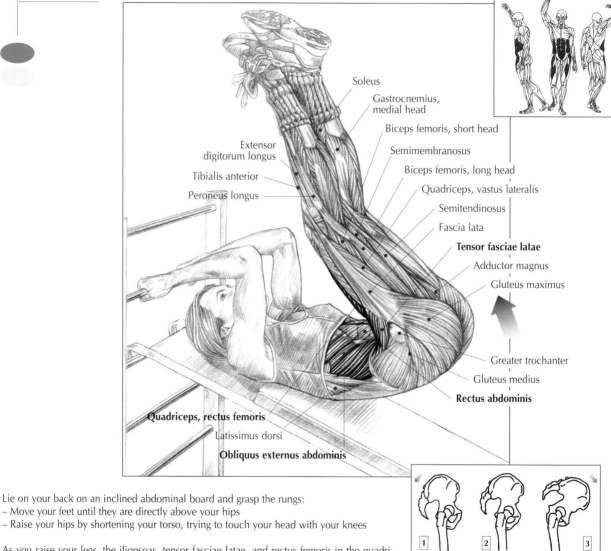

Soleus

Gastrocnemius, medial head

Biceps femoris, short head

Semimembranosus

Biceps femoris, long head

Quadriceps, vastus lateralis

Semitendinosus

Fascia lata

Tensor fasciae latae

Adductor magnus

Gluteus maximus

Greater trochanter

Gluteus medius

Rectus abdominis

Extensor digitorum longus

Tibialis anterior

Peroneus longus

Quadriceps, rectus femoris

Latissimus dorsi

Obliquus externus abdominis

Lie on your back on an inclined abdominal board and grasp the rungs:
– Move your feet until they are directly above your hips
– Raise your hips by shortening your torso, trying to touch your head with your knees

As you raise your legs, the iliopsoas, tensor fasciae latae, and rectus femoris in the quadriceps group are worked. Then, as you raise your hips and shorten your torso, the abdominals (particularly the rectus abdominis) are involved.

Pelvic movement : 1. backward tilting; 2. normal ; 3. forward tilting.

Note: this is an excellent exercise if you find it difficult to feel the work on your lower abdominals. Because this exercise is difficult, beginners should adjust the board to a lower angle.

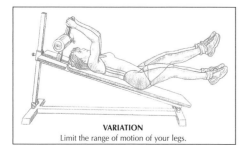

VARIATION
Limit the range of motion of your legs.

LEG RAISES 10

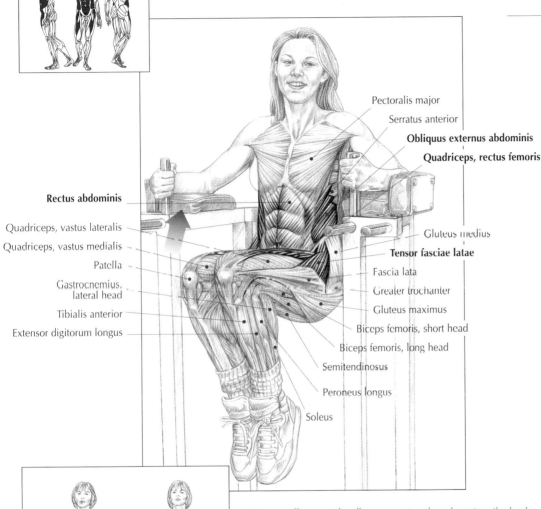

Pectoralis major

Serratus anterior

Obliquus externus abdominis

Quadriceps, rectus femoris

Rectus abdominis

Quadriceps, vastus lateralis

Quadriceps, vastus medialis

Patella

Gastrocnemius, lateral head

Tibialis anterior

Extensor digitorum longus

Gluteus medius

Tensor fasciae latae

Fascia lata

Greater trochanter

Gluteus maximus

Biceps femoris, short head

Biceps femoris, long head

Semitendinosus

Peroneus longus

Soleus

ACTION

Rest your elbows on the elbow support pads and position the lumbar support pad in the small of your back:

– Inhale and pull your knees up to your chest, rounding your back to contract your abdominals correctly
– Exhale as you complete the movement

This exercise works the hip flexors, particularly the iliopsoas, obliques, and rectus abdominis.

Variations:

1. To isolate the abdominals, limit the range of motion but never lower your knees to a position below the horizontal plane and always keep a slight curve in your spine.

2. To increase the difficulty of this movement, you can perform it with your legs straight. However, doing so requires flexible hamstrings.

3. You can hold the peak contracted position (knees tucked to chest) for a few seconds.

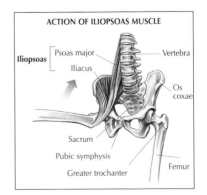

ACTION OF ILIOPSOAS MUSCLE

Iliopsoas

Psoas major

Iliacus

Vertebra

Os coxae

Sacrum

Pubic symphysis

Greater trochanter

Femur

11 HANGING LEG RAISES

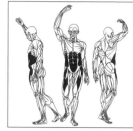

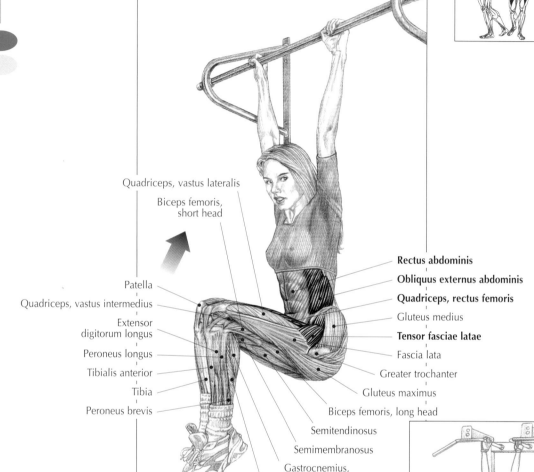

Quadriceps, vastus lateralis

Biceps femoris, short head

Patella

Quadriceps, vastus intermedius

Extensor digitorum longus

Peroneus longus

Tibialis anterior

Tibia

Peroneus brevis

Rectus abdominis

Obliquus externus abdominis

Quadriceps, rectus femoris

Gluteus medius

Tensor fasciae latae

Fascia lata

Greater trochanter

Gluteus maximus

Biceps femoris, long head

Semitendinosus

Semimembranosus

Gastrocnemius, lateral head

Soleus

Take an overhand grip on a chin-up bar. Hang straight.
– Inhale and raise your knees as high as possible, being sure to move your knees to your chest by shortening your torso
– Exhale as you complete the movement

This exercise works the following muscles:
– the iliopsoas, rectus femoris, and tensor fasciae latae as you raise your legs; and
– the rectus abdominis and, to a lesser extent, the obliques as you move your knees to your chest.

To isolate the abdominals, limit the range of motion, without lowering your knees to a position below the horizontal plane.

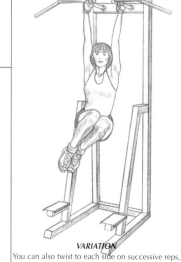

VARIATION
You can also twist to each side on successive reps, a movement which involves the obliques more intensely.

BROOMSTICK TWISTS **12**

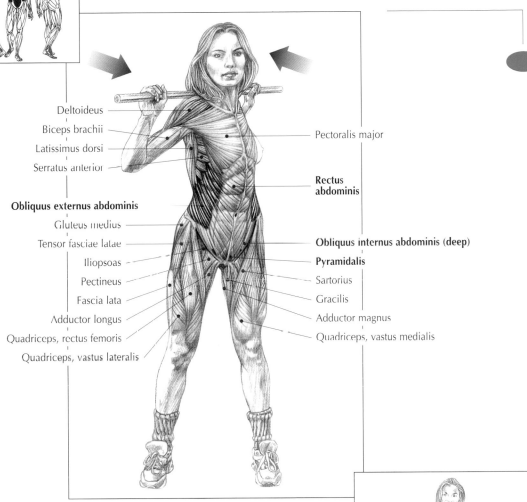

Deltoideus
Biceps brachii
Latissimus dorsi
Serratus anterior

Obliquus externus abdominis
Gluteus medius
Tensor fasciae latae
Iliopsoas
Pectineus
Fascia lata
Adductor longus
Quadriceps, rectus femoris
Quadriceps, vastus lateralis

Pectoralis major

Rectus abdominis

Obliquus internus abdominis (deep)
Pyramidalis
Sartorius
Gracilis
Adductor magnus
Quadriceps, vastus medialis

Stand with your feet spread. Hold a broomstick across your trapezius, above the posterior deltoids. Make sure you don't pull or hang too much on the broomstick:
– Rotate your upper body from side to side
– Keep your pelvis (hips) motionless by contracting the gluteals isometrically throughout the movement

As you rotate your right shoulder forward, this movement works the right external oblique, left internal oblique, and, to a lesser extent, the rectus abdominis and the left spinal erectors. To add intensity, you may slightly round your back. This exercise can also be done while sitting on a bench with your legs straddling the bench to keep your hips stationary and isolate the abdominals.

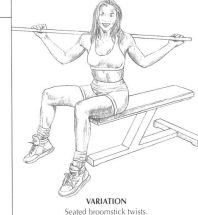

VARIATION
Seated broomstick twists.

13 DUMBBELL SIDE BENDS

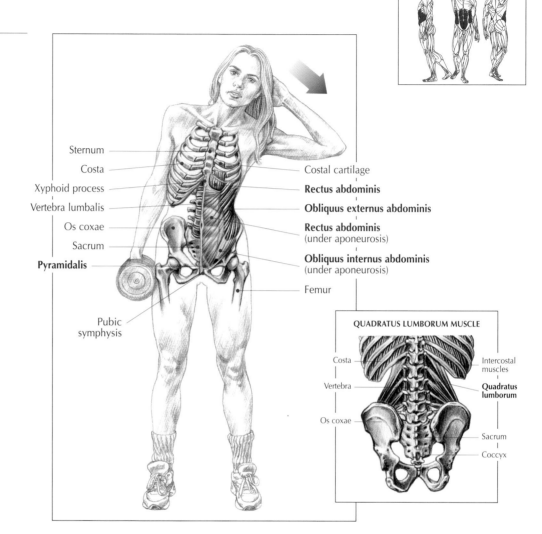

Sternum
Costa
Xyphoid process
Vertebra lumbalis
Os coxae
Sacrum
Pyramidalis

Costal cartilage
Rectus abdominis
Obliquus externus abdominis
Rectus abdominis
(under aponeurosis)
Obliquus internus abdominis
(under aponeurosis)
Femur

Pubic
symphysis

QUADRATUS LUMBORUM MUSCLE

Costa
Vertebra
Os coxae

Intercostal
muscles
**Quadratus
lumborum**
Sacrum
Coccyx

Stand with your feet slightly apart. Place your left hand behind your neck, holding a dumbbell in your right hand:
– Bend your torso to the left side
– Return to the starting position, or move slightly farther to the other side by bending at the waist passively

Be sure to do an equal number of sets and reps with the dumbbell held in each hand. Don't rest between the sets.
This exercise focuses on the obliques of the side you bend with and places secondary emphasis on the rectus abdominis and quadratus lumborum (muscle of the back attached to the 12th rib, transverse apophyses of the lumbar vertebrae, and crest of the shin).

ROMAN CHAIR SIDE BENDS 14

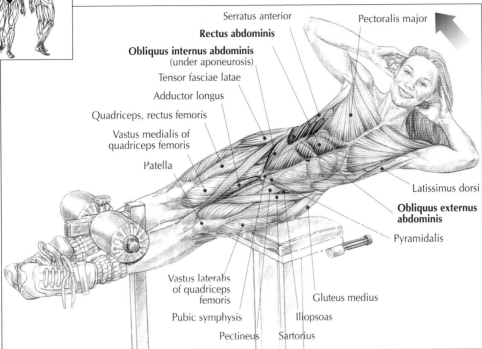

Serratus anterior
Pectoralis major
Rectus abdominis
Obliquus internus abdominis
(under aponeurosis)
Tensor fasciae latae
Adductor longus
Quadriceps, rectus femoris
Vastus medialis of
quadriceps femoris
Patella
Latissimus dorsi
**Obliquus externus
abdominis**
Pyramidalis
Vastus lateralis
of quadriceps
femoris
Gluteus medius
Pubic symphysis
Iliopsoas
Pectineus
Sartorius

Using a Roman chair, position your hip on the support pad. Hook your feet under the roller pads. Place your hands behind your head or across your chest, your upper body slightly above horizontal:
– Lift and twist your upper body upward
– Continue on the same side for one set, then alternate sides.

This movement focuses on the obliques and rectus abdominis of the side you bend, but the opposite obliques and rectus abdominis are also worked by contracting isometrically to prevent your torso from going below the horizontal plane.

Note: this movement continuously works the quadratus lumborum.

15 MACHINE TRUNK ROTATIONS

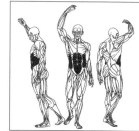

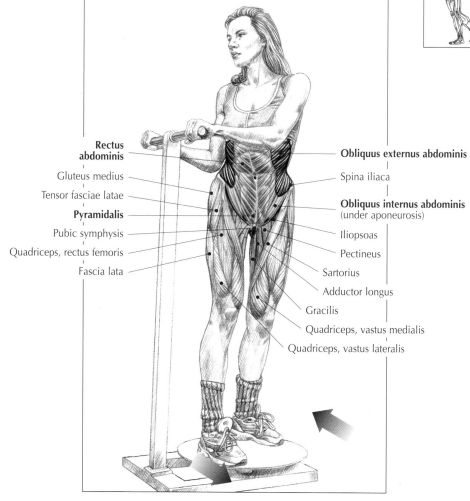

Rectus abdominis
Gluteus medius
Tensor fasciae latae
Pyramidalis
Pubic symphysis
Quadriceps, rectus femoris
Fascia lata

Obliquus externus abdominis
Spina iliaca
Obliquus internus abdominis
(under aponeurosis)
Iliopsoas
Pectineus
Sartorius
Adductor longus
Gracilis
Quadriceps, vastus medialis
Quadriceps, vastus lateralis

Stand on the swivel plate and hold the handles:
– Twist your hips from one side to the other being sure to keep your shoulders stationary throughout the movement
– Bend your knees slightly, making sure you perform this movement under control

This exercise works the external and internal obliques with secondary emphasis on the rectus abdominis. To feel the effort more strongly, you can slightly round your back.